The
Breast Cancer
Survival Manual

The

BREAST
CANCER

·SURVIVAL MANUAL·

A Step-by-Step Guide for Women
with Newly Diagnosed Breast Cancer

FIFTH EDITION

JOHN S. LINK, M.D.

WITH

JAMES WAISMAN, M.D.
NANCY LINK, R.D.

AN OWL BOOK
HENRY HOLT AND COMPANY · NEW YORK

Owl Books
Henry Holt and Company, LLC
Publishers since 1866
175 Fifth Avenue
New York, New York 10010

An Owl Book® and ® are registered trademarks of
Henry Holt and Company, LLC.

Library of Congress Cataloging-in-Publication Data

Breast cancer survival manual : a step-by-step guide for the woman with newly diagnosed
breast cancer / John S. Link . . . [et al.].—5th ed.
        p.   cm.
Rev. ed. of: Breast cancer survival manual / John Link, Cynthia Forsthoff, James Waisman.
Includes index.
ISBN 978-0-8050-9445-9
1. Breast—Cancer—Popular works.   I. Link, John S.   II. Link, John S. Breast cancer
survival manual.
RC280.B8L53 2012
616.99'449—dc23   2012017642

Henry Holt books are available for special promotions
and premiums. For details contact: Director, Special Markets.

First Owl Books Edition 1998
Second Owl Books Edition 2000
Third Owl Books Edition 2003
Fourth Owl Books Edition 2007
Fifth Owl Books Edition 2012

Designed by Victoria Hartman

Printed in the United States of America
3   5   7   9   10   8   6   4   2

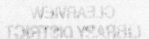

This book is dedicated to all of the women out there
who have stood strong and stared breast cancer dead in the eye,
fought it, and defied it!
I salute you.

Contents

❧

Acknowledgments

The *Breast Cancer Survival Manual* was conceived almost fourteen years ago as a teaching guide for women who came to my breast care center with newly diagnosed breast cancer. We had no idea the manual would receive such wide acclaim and acceptance. This fifth edition has required the most revision to date because of major advances in breast cancer diagnosis and treatment that have occurred over the past several years.

One of the most important lessons in this book is that optimal breast cancer care requires the collaboration of a team of dedicated breast specialists. I have had the privilege of working with and leading several outstanding breast cancer treatment teams in Southern California. I am deeply appreciative and grateful to my coauthor, good friend, and kindred spirit Dr. James Waisman, who shares my passion for the work we do. Our patients are so fortunate to have talented and dedicated breast surgeons led by Drs. John West, Helen Mabry, and Amy Bremner. We have a superb team of breast imagers led by Dr. June Chen and outstanding pathology under the guidance of Dr. Shu-Yuan Liao. I would like to thank Dr. Liao for providing images of breast cancer cell types as seen under the microscope that are included in this manual. I would like to thank Venita Williams, M.D., for her contribution to the chapter on radiation therapy.

Our breast care center in Orange, California, now includes a dedicated breast reconstruction surgeon, Dr. Justin West, and I want to acknowledge his expert contribution to the chapter on breast reconstruction techniques and options.

We could not provide the quality of care and service without a dedicated staff at all of our centers. I would like to especially acknowledge Donna Valentine, my physician assistant, for her commitment and dedication to the care of breast cancer patients. I would also like to acknowledge Stephanie Montalbano, Kami Levering, and Lisa Donely for their efforts on behalf of newly diagnosed women. Research is the key to progress, and we believe our patients should have access to the latest clinical trial protocols. I thank Cheryl Jacobs, research department manager, for her efforts in coordinating our research program.

I would especially like to thank my wife, Nancy Link, R.D., who made huge contributions to this edition of *The Breast Cancer Survival Manual*. In addition to her knowledge of nutrition and epidemiology, she has been my best critic, editor, and supporter; this edition would not have been possible without her tireless efforts.

I cannot bypass this opportunity to express gratitude to my parents, who raised me with love and gave me every opportunity to pursue my dreams. Both died far too early from this disease called cancer. My mother provided me with a wonderful New Zealand heritage and taught me to the last days of her life about hope and dignity. My father, a kind, gentle, and hardworking man, provided a brilliant example of how to live one's life with compassion and grace.

Heroes in my life who will always be an inspiration to me: my track coach at the University of Southern California, Willie Wilson, who died from cancer when I was nineteen years old, and my boyhood hero, Sir Edmund Hilary. Both of these gentlemen were the epitome of courage and dedication.

Last and most important, I would like to thank my patients, as they have taught me the most and are responsible for this book.

The
Breast Cancer
Survival Manual

Introduction

ABOUT THIS MANUAL

This book is a crisis manual. It is an attempt to put into writing the work we do on a daily basis, which is to help women with newly diagnosed breast cancer understand their situation and develop a plan to optimize a cure. With this life-altering and often life-threatening diagnosis, we ask women to become immediately educated and make critical decisions regarding their disease. We ask this at a time of immense crisis in a woman's life—a time of fear, confusion, and anxiety, and it doesn't seem fair. A newly diagnosed patient needs direct, useful, and honest information to help guide the choices she is being asked to make about the management of her cancer.

In our practice, we encounter women from all walks of life who have been given a diagnosis of breast cancer. Regardless of background, patients experience similar emotions, including shock, denial, fear, and a sense of urgency. Initially many patients lack the knowledge and information crucial for making sound decisions about medical care and are in no position to rush into treatment. This sense of urgency probably dates back to the old way of treating breast cancer, prior to 1970, when the *one-stage mastectomy*, or removal of the entire breast, underlying muscle, and axillary lymph nodes (also called radical mastectomy), was the only option. Treating breast cancer today involves a wide variety of options that may include surgery, radiation, chemotherapy, and/or hormones; the order and use of these treatments will vary depending on each woman's unique situation.

In the majority of cases, the diagnosis of breast cancer is based on the needle biopsy obtained prior to surgery. Needle biopsies can be performed on small, *nonpalpable* (cannot be felt) lesions using image-guided assistance with either an ultrasound machine or a mammogram. Palpable lesions that can be felt are also biopsied with a needle, so that a woman is usually fully aware of her cancer diagnosis *before* making the decision to undergo further surgical procedure.

One of the first and most important things we tell a patient in our clinic is that *she does have time*—usually several weeks to a month—in order to confirm the diagnosis, seek expert opinions, and develop a survival plan. By taking this extra time to establish the appropriate treatment plan, a woman will *not* decrease her chances of survival and may very well have an increased chance of cure. Taking a little time is very helpful because the course of therapy can be developed and implemented without *burning any bridges*. In other words, some treatment decisions made now cannot be undone later. Some patients will require limited surgery without the removal of lymph nodes in the *axilla* (armpit). In other cases women will need chemotherapy treatment before continuing on to a surgical procedure. Still others will receive radiation at the same time as they undergo surgery. There is no single treatment plan that is appropriate for all women with breast cancer, and taking the time to review and evaluate all available options will result in a tailored plan that is right for you.

The old method of treating women with breast cancer is what we call the sequential method, in which a woman sees a succession of independent specialists, usually beginning with the surgeon. Each physician will then do what his or her training dictates. For instance, the surgeon will operate, then the radiation oncologist will give radiation therapy, and finally the oncologist will administer chemotherapy. This sequential approach is not always well coordinated and can lead to duplication and overtreatment or delay in treatment due to a lack of communication and proper sequencing.

Today's newer approach to breast cancer diagnosis and treatment integrates all of the treating specialists into a single team. The optimal care of breast cancer involves the breast surgeon, plastic surgeon, radiation oncologist, medical oncologist, pathologist, and radiologist, working closely together and coordinated by a team leader. The team leader could be any one of your treating doctors, but there must be mutual understanding that this physician is assuming the role. Clearly, this is what any patient wants: the various treating physicians communicating with one another and working toward a unified treatment plan designed with each individual woman in mind.

At our breast care centers, once a breast cancer diagnosis has been established and we have collected the necessary information from imaging, pathology, and gene testing, our *treatment planning team* meets to develop a *treatment plan* designed for each woman. The treatment team includes the patient's primary caregiver, breast surgeon, reconstruction/plastic surgeon, radiologist, pathologist, and the medical oncologist, as well as nurses, social workers, and other medical support staff as needed. Weekly meetings, or *treatment planning conferences*, allow the entire team the opportunity to review every case together as a group and make collaborative recommendations. The *diagnostic team* presents the radiologic images, and the *pathology team* provides information about how the cancer appears under the microscope. The *treatment team* then develops a plan based on each patient's individual cancer situation. This team also evaluates each woman's eligibility for one of the currently enrolling clinical research trials. Once the options, recommendations, and potential research protocols have been identified during the pretreatment planning conference, one of the treating physicians will present this information to the patient and her own personal support team.

Armed with the recommended treatment plan, the newly diagnosed woman is now ready to begin the tailored treatment protocol or to do further research, possibly seeking a second opinion. Many breast care centers today utilize treatment planning conferences, and you may want to search out a center that includes such a program.

With recent changes in health care delivery, women may have difficulty finding someone who can coordinate their care. In a managed care system, choices may differ from the private-practice model. If you are in a health maintenance organization (HMO), you can receive "state-of-the-art" therapy, but it is critical that you become well educated and play a leading role in directing your care. You may need to go outside your HMO for a second opinion. Some managed care organizations will pay for this, although it may take some assertiveness on your part to obtain approval. Getting a second opinion may add an extra week before actual treatment can begin, but *it will be time well spent.*

As stated previously, we would like to strongly emphasize that breast cancer is unique in every woman. Breast cancer has a tremendous variability in the way it comes into existence, the way it looks under the microscope, the way it behaves biologically, and the way it interacts *within* each individual woman. These factors are extremely important in planning therapy.

In the past the medical profession tended to simplify breast cancer and make it all the same, or *homogeneous*, so that treatment could be standardized for all women. Although we know that breast cancer has a number of commonalities, we now know this does not justify using the same treatment for every woman. We've come a long way since the 1950s, when the only treatment for breast cancer was a radical mastectomy. We have a much better understanding of how to manage cancer within the breast (*local control*) and the factors that affect the cancer's ability to spread into the lymph and blood systems (*systemic control*). Our current knowledge base and technological development now allow us to treat breast cancer using an individualized approach, which is more effective for you and your particular cancer situation.

Clearly, we must identify each woman's unique cancer profile in order to make the best treatment choices. This profile allows us to look at a number of characteristics, including size of the tumor, type of cell, growth behavior of the cancer, influence of hormones, ability to attract and invade lymph and blood vessels, and genetic changes. Understanding genetic changes has led to new and better treatments and outcomes. Since the last edition of this book, this is where the most progress has been made. But don't worry; this is not as complex as it may sound to you now. Most of this information is available from your mammograms and your tissue biopsy, and you will have a much better understanding of how to interpret your own unique cancer profile after reading this manual.

It would be a tremendous mistake to treat breast cancer without considering the woman herself. A woman's age, hormone status, general health, emotional support network, sexuality, immune system, and psychological and spiritual being are all extremely important in planning treatment and maintaining health. Because traditional medicine often seems to neglect treating the whole person, many women today seek *complementary therapy* outside mainstream medicine. A few women are so distrustful of traditional medical treatment that they choose to rely exclusively on alternative therapies. Unfortunately, when some of these women come back to conventional medicine months to years later, they have more advanced breast cancer and are in a state of crisis. The treating physician should address the benefits of nutrition, vitamins and other supplements, psychotherapy, and physical therapy, in conjunction with state-of-the-art conventional therapy.

Chapter 1 of this manual begins your breast cancer education with a discussion about the nature and biology of breast cancer and how this affects your overall treatment plan. In today's world, where knowledge is power, a woman who is well informed has increased confidence in her diagnosis and treatment plan and becomes her own advocate and partner with her treating team. Selection of an appropriate treatment team is critical to achieving optimal breast cancer care. We also believe that keeping track of your health history will help you to be an active and informed participant in your care and survival. We encourage you to manage your personal health information using a format that is best suited to you. In chapter 2 we provide important tips on how to choose your treatment team, obtain a second opinion, and collect and store your own comprehensive health records.

Determining your breast cancer type will help your medical team determine the best treatment for you. In chapter 3 we present the types or classifications of breast cancer currently used. Accurate interpretation of what your cancer looks like under the microscope is absolutely critical to define your specific breast cancer type and develop the tailored treatment plan. In chapter 4, we discuss in depth how to analyze your pathology report and the importance and use of this information in planning your optimal care. Chapter 5 is devoted to ductal carcinoma in situ (DCIS), an early cancer that accounts for up to 20 percent of newly diagnosed breast cancers, while chapter 6 addresses the remaining 80 percent of women, those who have been diagnosed with invasive breast cancer.

Throughout this manual, we will emphasize obtaining optimal treatment for your particular cancer. If you are overtreated, you may suffer unnecessary side effects or even physical complications. On the other hand, if you're undertreated, you may face a more devastating prospect: being denied the latest and most up-to-date treatment and the best chance of being cured. In chapters 7 and 8 we discuss the most current treatment options.

Some women will require radiation therapy to prevent local recurrence. In chapter 9 we discuss the indications for inclusion of radiation as well as the different delivery methods. Chapter 10 addresses the management of treatment-induced side effects. For women who require mastectomy or significant removal of breast tissue, chapter 11 covers breast reconstruction and the current innovations that are changing women's attitudes toward this previously feared procedure.

Much scientific advancement in breast cancer treatment occurring over the last few years is a result of patients enrolling in clinical research trials. In chapter 12 we discuss the clinical trial research process and how women can participate.

We now know that a small percentage of women are predisposed to breast cancer and carry a gene that they inherited from one of their parents that increases the risk of breast or ovarian cancer. Genetics and the criteria for genetic testing are explored in chapter 13. In this chapter we provide resources to help you understand and create your own family health pedigree.

Over the next few months you will be consumed with your breast cancer diagnosis and treatment, but you then will go on as a breast cancer survivor, which will affect how you live the rest of your life. Chapters 14 and 15 address lifestyle choices and issues, including nutrition, exercise, sexuality, and quality of life.

It is our hope that this manual will be helpful to you during a difficult period. Over the past fourteen years our medical practice has been devoted to women with breast cancer, and we have seen the positive effects of patient participation in forming the treatment plan. Since more and more physicians today are asking for their patients' input on important decisions regarding treatment, having proper preparation to become an informed participant will empower you to participate in the decision-making process. Keep in mind that most women are fearful that their recommended therapy could be inadequate. Of equal concern, however, is overtreatment. Many women are being overtreated without understanding the true risks, benefits, and appropriateness of the therapy they receive. We hope to help alleviate these fears by clearly describing all of the options available to you and directing you to resources where you can get more answers.

The main objective of this book is to educate you about breast cancer and to give you some control over what may now seem like chaos. Information and knowledge are critical and constantly changing. You have access to the latest information on breast cancer diagnosis and treatment through numerous resources, including your medical team, support groups, a wide variety of printed material, and the Internet; see the Resources section at the back of the book for a number of important Web sites. Although we have updated the information contained in this manual on a continuing basis (now in our fifth edition), the process stops at the time of publication. To provide you with the latest in breast cancer research, diagnosis, and treatment, we invite you to visit us at http://www.breastlink.com.

We recommend that you use this manual as your breast cancer treatment workbook. Keep notes and highlight important information. As we describe in chapter 2, you may want to begin tracking your own personal health history by collecting and managing copies of your medical records. This can be accomplished using a three-ring binder or electronically on your computer. There are several different personal health record applications available on the Internet and you can select the one best for you. In addition we have created a breast cancer specific medical records tool that may be helpful for this purpose. It is available at http://www.drjohnlink.com.

Whether you skim *The Breast Cancer Survival Manual* once or it never leaves your side throughout treatment, we hope it will inform and empower you, helping you to receive the breast cancer treatment and care that is *right for you* during this challenging time in your life.

1
· · · · · ·

Breast Cancer Basics

can•cer *noun* \'kan(t)-sər\ : a malignant tumor of potentially unlimited growth that expands locally by invasion and systemically by metastasis

Before beginning our discussion about cancer of the breast, I want to give you some very basic information about cancer in general and how its unique characteristics compare to a normal cell.

Normal body cells can:

- Reproduce themselves EXACTLY
- Stop reproducing at the right moment
- Stick together in the correct place
- Self-destruct if a mistake occurs or they are damaged
- Mature and become specialized
- Die (they are programmed to do so), and when appropriate they are renewed by *like* cells

Cancer cells are different from normal cells in the following ways:

- Cancer cells don't stop reproducing
- Cancer cells don't obey signals from other cells
- Cancer cells don't stick together; they can break off and float away
- Cancer cells stay immature and don't specialize, so they become more and more primitive, and they reproduce quickly and haphazardly
- Cancers cells lose their programmed death pathway

In this chapter we are going to explore the nature of breast cancer. It is a mystery to us why the female breast is vulnerable to developing cancer. It may have something to do with monthly cycling of glandular cells, yet more than half of breast cancers develop in older women after the breast glands have come to rest. We know that cancer tends to occur in organs with cells that are constantly cycling through cell renewal. The replacement of a cell requires the production of a new set of genes, and this process can lead to mistakes (*mutations*) that the cell is unable to repair. The mistakes can then be repeated, causing a cell to grow according to a new blueprint in a process that is out of control, and this process results in cancer.

First, let's examine the anatomy of the female breast (Figure 1.1). The female breast is composed of milk-producing *lobules* connected to milk *ducts* that carry milk from the lobule to the nipple. There are at least twelve or more of these separate branching ductal-lobular units that occupy the four quadrants of the breast. Supporting and surrounding the glandular units are fibrous tissue, fat cells, blood vessels, and the lymphatic system that drains from the breast to the lymph nodes. We believe that the majority of breast cancers are due to a genetic mistake within the cells lining the *lobules* or *ducts*. There is evidence that genetic mistakes are common, and the majority are harmless. Cells actually have the ability to self-repair these genetic mistakes so that they do not go on to become cancer.

A cancer is born when a mistake occurs at a critical point in the

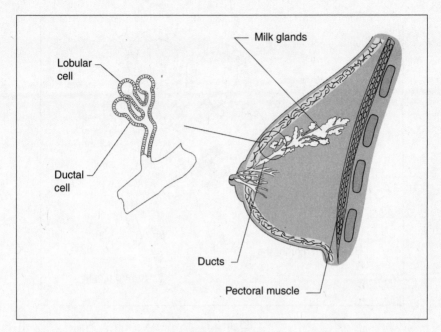

Figure 1.1
Breast ducts and lobules

cell's genetic blueprint, or *DNA*, and it goes unrepaired. This genetic mistake affects the behavior and characteristics of the affected cell and the new cells that are produced. When a cell becomes genetically unstable, it has gone bad. These unstable cells continue to divide, passing along the damaged or mutant genetic message to the next generation of cells.

As the new cluster of cancer cells emerges from a milk duct or lobule in the breast, it can remain within the duct system (*in situ*), or it can invade the basement membrane and spread into the fat and supporting tissue (*invasive or infiltrating*). (See Figure 1.2.) This ability to grow and invade is a characteristic of cancer, and it can spread locally, within the breast, or spread into lymph and blood vessels.

The resulting group of cancerous cells (*clone*) can have most of the same characteristics as the normal breast duct cell (i.e., hormone receptors) and grow slowly but steadily. On the other hand, the mutation(s)

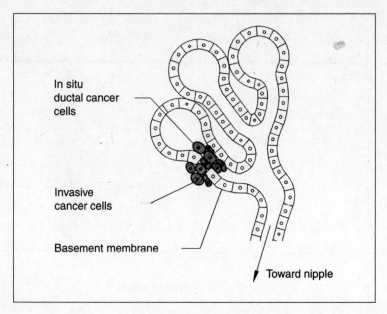

Figure 1.2

In situ and invasive ductal cancer

can lead to a clone that is highly malignant, with the resulting cells having no resemblance to the normal breast cells. We are beginning to understand that not all breast cancers are alike; they behave differently depending on the type of mutation and the resulting proteins or lack of proteins that direct the cell's behavior.

We now have the ability to analyze genetic material within cancer cells and map the unique patterns. From this research a new method of classifying breast cancer has emerged (see the discussion in chapter 3).

Breast cancers can remain contained within the duct system (in situ) for months or even years. Some cancers may require an additional mistake (mutation) to invade into the surrounding tissue. Other cancers probably immediately invade the surrounding tissue with the initial mutation. Cancers that remain in the duct system are called *ductal carcinoma in situ* (DCIS). (We discuss these preinvasive cancers in chapter 5.) If we can discover a DCIS before it invades the surrounding tissue, there is no risk of its spreading to the body, and the cancer is highly curable with local treatment measures.

The rate of growth of a cancer varies considerably and is very dependent on the mutation that has occurred. Some breast cancers retain the ability to be influenced by hormones (estrogen), and the presence or lack of estrogen will influence their growth.

The genetic blueprint (DNA) within a cancer cell is unstable, and with continued growth further mutations occur. Some of these mutations are so unstable that they become lethal to the cell population itself, thus ending the cancer growth. We tend to think of cancers as "strong" rogue cells. In reality many cancer cells, especially the most malignant, are fragile and just hanging on. Current treatments are able to take advantage of this fragile state, and in the future treatments will target this vulnerability.

As stated earlier, the rate of growth of breast cancer cells varies considerably. The slower growing cancers of the Luminal A type (see chapter 3) take six or more months to double in size (Figure 1.3), while the triple-negative (basal cell) cancers can double in size in just one to two months. The ability to spread into the lymph system and bloodstream depends on the underlying DNA mutation and the size of the cancer. Most cancers cannot spread into lymph and blood vessels (*metastasis*) until they exceed about 1 centimeter (10 mm) in size (Figure 1.4). We believe that over time slower-growing cancers can further

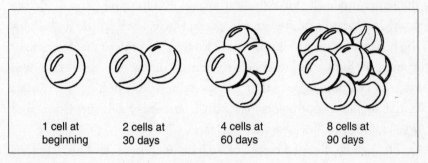

| 1 cell at beginning | 2 cells at 30 days | 4 cells at 60 days | 8 cells at 90 days |

Figure 1.3
Growth of cancer cells over time

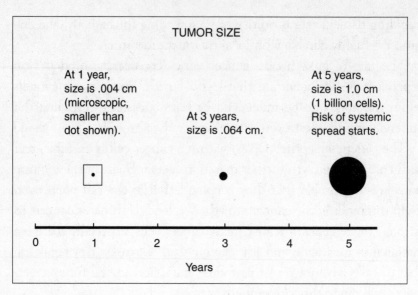

Figure 1.4

Tumor growth over time of a luminal breast cancer

mutate and increase their growth rate, potential to spread, and degree of malignancy.

Once a cancer has become invasive, there is risk of its spreading into the lymphatic system and the bloodstream. We are not sure what mechanism a cancer cell uses to invade vessels, but it is thought that the process requires DNA programming or mutation. Women often ask if a needle biopsy can disrupt cells and cause them to spread into the lymph nodes. I think this can occur, and in some cases we do see *isolated tumor cells* shortly after biopsy in the *first lymph node* that drains the breast. But we also know these women have the same outcome as women without the presence of isolated tumor cells in their lymph nodes. Evidence suggests that the spread to the lymph by the trauma of the biopsy is not associated with true cancer cell metastasis and does not lead to a decrease in cure rates.

The needle-directed biopsy of a cancer is the standard for diagnosis of breast cancer. From this small core of tissue, about the size of a pencil lead, the type of breast cancer can be determined, allowing the treatment team to plan therapy most appropriate for the patient. (We discuss the analysis of tumor tissue more completely in chapter 4.)

In the past we placed huge importance in staging a cancer on analysis of the draining lymph nodes, looking for spread of tumor cells and extent of the spread. Figure 1.5 demonstrates the distribution of lymph nodes draining the breast. Until a few years ago surgeons would remove a majority of the lymph nodes at the time of the breast cancer surgery. Spread to lymph nodes is an important factor to determine your *prognosis* (probable course or outcome of the disease), but it is no longer necessary to do extensive lymph node surgery. There is increased risk of *lymphedema* (arm swelling) that does not justify the information gained through removal of the majority of nodes. Instead, by removing

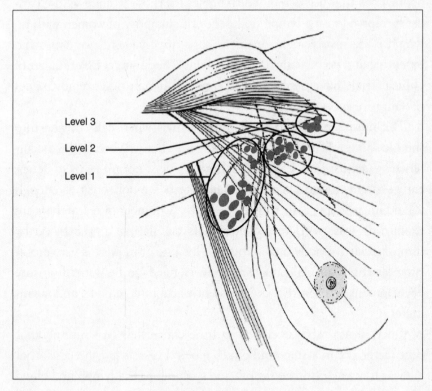

Figure 1.5
Distribution of axillary lymph nodes

the *sentinel node* (the first draining lymph node; see chapter 6), we can obtain the needed information without the risks of more extensive surgery. If there is extensive lymph node involvement at the time of diagnosis, the involved lymph nodes are usually treated with systemic therapy, followed by radiation and in some cases surgery.

Historically, lymph node involvement was the strongest predictor of risk of spread into the bloodstream. This is changing. Using a number of tests that can be performed on the needle biopsy, we have greatly improved our ability to assess the risk of cancer spread. (This topic is discussed further in chapters 4 and 6.)

It is important to treat cancer in the lymph nodes draining from the breast. By using sentinel lymph node sampling, ultrasound, and other imaging techniques such as MRI and PET scans, we can plan approaches that use combined therapies for those women whose cancer has spread to the lymph nodes. For the majority of women with no lymph node involvement or microscopic involvement, we can avoid extensive and potentially damaging lymph node surgery. A number of clinical trials have demonstrated that full lymph node removal *does not* improve survival rates.

The most serious and dangerous event is when cells invade into the blood vessels and metastasize into the body. We call this occurrence *systemic spread*. Current technology does not allow us to detect early systemic disease because imaging tests are not sensitive enough to find microscopic cells within the body. A number of researchers are examining ways to detect cancer cells circulating in the blood by using special antibody preparations. This line of inquiry is very promising for the future, although more work needs to be done to ensure development of a test that is consistently accurate, reliable, and meaningful.

Once invasion has occurred and the cancer has grown to about 1 centimeter, it can attract and produce blood vessels (*angiogenesis*) that allow it to break off (*metastasize*) and spread into the lymph and blood system (systemic spread). In this critical process, the cancer cells produce protein messengers known as *vascular endothelial growth factors*

(VegF). To counteract the effects of VegF, researchers have developed a number of antibodies and molecules that can reduce or prevent angiogenesis and ultimately lead to the destruction of the cancer.

With new technologies such as *reverse transcription-polymerase chain reaction* (RT-PCR), researchers are able to compare the genetic blueprint of a normal cell to the transformed malignant cell and identify the abnormal mutant genes. Identification of abnormal gene patterns has led to a new classification (*typing*) system for breast cancer that will be discussed in chapter 3. This ability to analyze the mutant genes has also led to the recognition that certain of the abnormalities are related to cancer cell functions such as invasion, proliferation (cell growth), angiogenesis, and metastasis.

Using these techniques, commercial laboratories have been able to analyze cancer cells for the presence of mutant genes associated with systemic spread and to develop tests that can predict how likely a cancer is to recur or metastasize. Several of these *prognostic* (predictors) tests have been developed by two labs: Genomic Health in Northern California, which has a twenty-one-gene test called Oncotype DX; and Agendia in Irvine, California, which has a seventy-gene test known as MammaPrint. Both tests help the cancer specialist to select those women who may benefit from systemic therapies.

Based on the identification of gene mutations, it is now possible to develop therapies targeted at the specific mutations; these therapies can reverse the effects of these mutations and potentially reverse the malignant process. In the previous edition of this book, I alluded to this possibility, which has now become a reality.

2

The Launchpad

KNOWLEDGE IS POWER & SECOND OPINIONS

You may feel frightened and overwhelmed at this point, which is not unusual. When I see a newly diagnosed patient, I tell her that the chance of being cured (yes, cured!) is very high. You do have time to educate yourself, gather information, and even obtain a second opinion if desired. Just remember, take one step at a time! Let me show you how.

The modern diagnosis of breast cancer is made with a needle biopsy following an abnormal mammogram or after a lump is discovered, typically by you, your spouse or partner, or your physician. At this point women often feel a tremendous urgency to have the breast cancer surgically removed RIGHT NOW! It bears repeating: you do have time to gather information and decide on a comprehensive and appropriate treatment plan.

There have been tremendous advancements in our understanding of breast cancer in recent years. We now know that breast cancer is not the same in every woman; it is different, or *heterogeneous*. The more we learn about the nature of breast cancer, the more effective and targeted the therapy we can recommend, and the greater chance you will receive the appropriate care. In most cases optimal treatment planning can be done effectively with comprehensive imaging and needle biopsy prior to embarking on any major surgery. With modern imaging using mammography, ultrasound, and MRI, we can accurately determine the size and extent of the cancer. Carefully examining the cancer tissue biopsy under the microscope, we can learn a great deal about your specific cancer, that is, the cell type, the different receptors on the cell surface, and how aggressive the malignancy is. (We will explain all of this thoroughly in the next several chapters.) Armed with as much information as we can gather about your cancer, we are able to establish the most effective treatment options.

Interestingly, in spite of advancements in our understanding of breast cancer, the fundamentals of treatment have not changed significantly over time. We continue to be governed by the concepts of *local control* and *systemic control*. Here is a brief explanation of these two very important concepts in cancer treatment. (Chapter 6 provides a detailed discussion of this topic.)

- *Local control* is achieved by mapping the location of the cancer in the breast and lymph nodes and then using appropriate and effective treatments to eliminate it before it has had a chance to spread beyond its place of origin.
- If there is a chance that cancer cells have escaped from the original tumor into the rest of the body (the *system*), these cells must also be eliminated in a process referred to as *systemic control*.

Women start this journey in different medical systems. Regardless of the medical system you are in, you are still able to receive coordinated care. The ultimate goal is to survive the cancer with the least amount of side effect and disability.

The United States is currently struggling to reformulate our health care system. As it stands in 2012, women covered by traditional insurance plans have access to physicians and specialists of their own choosing. The alternative system limits patient choices to a group of physicians and specialists who are members of an organized group. You can get excellent care in both types of health care systems, but this will require education, understanding, and oversight on your part. Both systems have their own advantages and disadvantages.

Traditional Fee-for-Service Health Insurance Model

- A newly diagnosed patient has the freedom to access individual doctors who are in private practice. This allows the patient to seek out potential specialists of her own choosing based on reputation, recommendation, or referral.
- The patient can seek out and select a surgeon or oncologist who specializes primarily in breast cancer.
- Another plus is the patient's access to cutting-edge, outside-the-box treatments.
- One disadvantage of this system is that there is no guarantee that the selected specialists will work together as a treatment team or that they will work within a system of collaborative management. The risk is that decision-making will be made independent of the other treating specialists without development of a comprehensive plan.
- There is also no guarantee that the independent specialists will work together toward a coordinated treatment plan, or that one of them will be responsible for performing the job of team leader.

Managed Care Health Insurance Model

- The main advantage of a managed care system is that specific guidelines are most likely in place, including planning and treatment conferences and established protocols for breast cancer diagnosis and treatment. This can ensure consistency in diagnostic and treatment regimens through standardized procedures.
- Another advantage in some cases is the sharing of electronic medical records databases, which allows all treatment team members to easily follow treatment activities and for ongoing review of the quality of care and analysis of outcomes.

- One disadvantage is that patients are usually locked into the system and cannot go outside it for treatment.
- There is often some restriction on use of cutting-edge drugs or technology until there is absolute scientific evidence to support it from a cost-benefit perspective. In no way does this mean that someone cannot get excellent care in this type of system. (In fact, premature use of new technology may not always lead to a better outcome.)
- There may not be access to surgeons or oncologists who specialize exclusively in breast cancer.

Regardless of the system you are in, your understanding of and involvement in your health care are equally important, and you should feel empowered to advocate on your own behalf. This might involve obtaining additional knowledge and education (this manual is a good place to start) or obtaining a second opinion.

Now that your cancer diagnosis has been confirmed, by needle biopsy or abnormal mammogram, and the extent of the cancer has been established by breast and lymph node imaging, the next step is to select your treatment team.

Picking the Treatment Team and Coordinating Care

The diagnosis and treatment of breast cancer have changed dramatically over the past thirty years. Back then a majority of women who had a palpable breast lump went directly into surgery. Often the operation was a mastectomy, and that was the full extent of their treatment. Researchers were just beginning to explore the role of *adjuvant chemotherapy*, and *radiation* was a new kind of treatment utilized by a few brave women.

Today, the majority of breast cancers are discovered by mammography. These cancers are small, often too small to be felt, and surgeons rely on radiologists to find or *localize* them with a hook wire or injected blue dye. As you can see, the technology has changed dramatically, and we have entered a new era of breast cancer diagnosis and therapy. Because of the many elements that come into play in cancer diagnosis and treatment, good coordination is critical among a team of physicians: surgeon, radiologist, pathologist, radiation oncologist, plastic surgeon, and medical oncologist.

Ideally, a woman with a newly diagnosed breast cancer connects with a key physician who takes charge for developing a treatment plan with her and who then coordinates the implementation of the plan with the other team members. The group of physicians can work at a single institution or be drawn from a wider geographic area, and any of the cancer specialists can act as the coordinating doctor. At our center, it is usually the medical oncologist who coordinates the flow of information and treatment for a patient, but our surgeons and radiation oncologists can take on this pivotal role as well.

We hope you will find a cancer specialist you can communicate with comfortably and who will address your concerns. However, there are medical systems in which it may be difficult for the patient to connect with one physician who will act as the coordinating team leader. If this describes your situation, don't despair. This manual will give you some information and suggestions to help you function as your own team leader. It is possible to go through this process without a physician to spearhead your treatment plan and still receive state-of-the-art care.

The overall treatment plan revolves around two critical decisions. The first deals with *local control* and the second with the need for *systemic adjuvant therapy*. Often you and your doctors cannot decide upon the issue of systemic therapy until all the information is available from the needle biopsy or from the surgical procedure.

Since the diagnosis and treatment of breast cancer is achieved primarily in an outpatient setting, you may travel to various locations for different aspects of your care. In our community, some women come to our center for surgery and then have radiation at a facility closer to their home. If you require various therapies, you may want to consider coordinating something similar in order to make your treatment appointments as convenient as possible.

From your first decision about whom to contact for your breast cancer care all the way through the many follow-up exams after your treatment is completed, communication is key. Establish a relationship with a physician that will enable you to develop an overall treatment plan that will flow as smoothly as possible. You should also get to know the nurses and other medical staff well. Nurse specialists often play very important roles by coordinating and facilitating the communication process between you and your doctors.

At our centers, one of the key tools used in coordinating a woman's care is the *treatment planning conference.* This conference is a meeting of the medical team members to discuss each patient's case and to develop a coordinated treatment plan. The conference allows all team members to review the health history, radiological breast images, pathology report, and pathology slides. The patient does not participate in the treatment planning conference.

After the conference you should be apprised of the process and the conclusions reached by the team. Some centers actually give patients formal minutes or written conclusions. Other centers arrange for the conclusions to be verbally presented to you by the team member who is coordinating your care. Usually, the discussion and recommendations made at the pretreatment planning conference are shared with you by the physician who presented your case at the group meeting.

The treatment planning conference is extremely important in coordinating care. Each of the potential treating physicians can, in one setting, agree on an overall treatment plan and his or her particular contribution to that plan. This united approach also guarantees that the doctors line up the sequencing of the different therapies correctly and in the manner that is most beneficial to the overall well-being of the patient. The conference also allows us to identify women who are eligible for special research studies and protocols sponsored by the government or other research groups. At our centers this important aspect provides our patients with state-of-the-art care and promotes medical advancement.

Besides benefiting the individual woman with breast cancer, the nature of the conference promotes education and understanding on the part of the various physicians involved. Younger or new physicians and those in training are often invited to attend the treatment planning conference. This is an invaluable experience as they are exposed to a wide variety of patients and situations, which would otherwise take years to accomplish in their own practices. In addition, women diagnosed in the future will benefit greatly from the wealth of knowledge that these conferences provide medical professionals.

Seeking a Second Opinion

Once the treatment team has been selected, many women find it helpful to seek a second opinion so that they have confidence in the diagnosis and treatment plan before commencing with the chosen course of action. It is important for us to note that many women and their families feel anxious or guilty about asking the diagnosing physician to help them gather materials and records to give to another physician or institution for a second opinion. *You don't need to worry about this.* It has become such a common practice that physicians are neither surprised nor insulted by such requests.

There are several important reasons to get a second opinion when you have been diagnosed with breast cancer. Even when you trust your physicians completely, the gravity of a cancer diagnosis demands that you feel fully confident with the diagnosis and treatment plan before proceeding any further. A second opinion that concurs with the first opinion can give you that confidence. Although confirmation is reassuring, a second opinion can also add to or conflict with information you have already received. Remember that both *conflicting* and *confirming* data will help establish productive dialogue that can lead to a more appropriate treatment plan and a better understanding of your unique situation.

You might think that breast cancer is so common that the recommended treatment must be fairly standard among doctors. This was more true twenty years ago, when our understanding of breast cancer was much less sophisticated and the treatment options were limited. Current treatment involves a wealth of new tests, *agents* (medicines), and procedures. You want to receive the very best that medicine can offer today, with treatment options tailored specifically for you and your diagnosis.

We diagnose hundreds of women with breast cancer every year. We also render hundreds of second opinions to women with newly diagnosed breast cancer who come to us from a number of other facilities around the United States and around the world. Even though we are regarded as experts in the field, we understand a woman's need to hear confirmation from another source. In any way we can, we encourage and facilitate obtaining a second opinion for any patient. We feel it is extremely important that every woman be comfortable with and have confidence in her treatment team. We welcome outside opinions before embarking on a course of therapy. Occasionally, new information is brought forth from another source, or a different approach is presented that is better suited to the patient. Do not be afraid or hesitant about requesting a second opinion; your doctor should not be concerned about your receiving one. On the contrary, this process is usually encouraged, and any center or physician that discourages a second opinion should be willing to discuss their reasons with you for not supporting this very important issue.

A thorough, comprehensive second opinion takes time and may be expensive—between $500 and $1,000. (Some insurance plans pay for second opinions.) It includes an independent review of the biopsy tissue by a pathologist, a review of x-rays and imaging studies by a breast radiologist, and presentation to a treatment team for review and recommendations for a treatment plan. This process requires the integration of a team of experienced experts. The second opinion is usually enlightening, confirming information you already obtained from your diagnosing doctor and from your own independent research.

Occasionally, the second opinion differs drastically from the first, placing you in a dilemma. If the institution rendering the differing opinion is experienced and reputable, the medical team will explain the basis of their opinion to you and your diagnosing physicians. You might ask how, in this age of modern medicine, can there be a major difference in opinion about managing an individual's breast cancer. In our experience, the most common recommendations provided by our second opinions have to do with women not receiving coordinated care. In many cases we point out overlaps, delays, and overtreatment.

Breast cancer testing and treatment are constantly evolving, and occasionally physicians may be practicing *older*—out of date—medicine. Newer treatments are often targeted directly at the cancer and are therefore less toxic for the rest of the body. New tools and genetic analysis help us plan appropriate, optimal treatment, but some physicians may not be utilizing all available technologies. Finally, while a mistake in the initial diagnosis is rare, a review of the actual biopsy tissue and of the radiologic images is a must. Sometimes a third opinion is necessary when there is a major difference between your first and second opinions. This should be rendered by a center that specializes in breast cancer treatment. In our practice we sometimes see women who are seeking a fourth or even a fifth opinion. Additional opinions beyond the third will usually differ little and will only delay your decision regarding a treatment plan and the commencement of treatment.

Differences in opinion may affect your medical outcome, or they may be as minor as a different sequencing of therapy (the order in which you receive treatments). A second opinion may propose a different type of chemotherapy, radiation, or hormone therapy, but with a very similar medical outcome to that predicted in the first opinion. Some recommendations may lead to different side effects or affect their duration, experiences which are much less critical and do not affect survival. The point is there may be differences in opinion, and some are minor and some are major.

Frequently encountered differences in opinion

1. Extent of breast surgery—mastectomy versus *partial mastectomy* (breast conservation)
2. Extent of lymph node sampling
3. Need for radiation combined with surgery
4. Risks and/or benefits of systemic treatment
5. Sequencing of systemic treatment and surgery

There may also be a variety of more subtle differences regarding radiation therapy, chemotherapy, or hormone therapy. The type and intensity of the therapy selected will depend to a large extent on the availability of new technologies within a medical system and of existing research protocols that may have unproven benefit versus risk to the patient. Just because it's new doesn't always mean it's better! *New* becomes better only after scientific confirmation, followed by government review and approval as a standard therapy. Women diagnosed with breast cancer can consider participating in a clinical trial (the focus of chapter 12).

You should start the process of obtaining a second opinion as soon as possible after you make the decision to seek one. Your diagnosing doctor may be helpful in recommending a physician or facility that specializes in breast cancer treatment, such as a university, a large urban hospital, or a private facility. The process of securing another doctor's or team's opinion involves several steps and may take a week or more to complete. We believe the best second opinion for women with newly diagnosed breast cancer is multidisciplinary and requires a thorough review of imaging and pathology, so be sure you provide complete documentation from your diagnosis. The following items will be needed: (1) copies of all breast imaging, including mammograms, ultrasounds, or MRI (if an image-guided biopsy was performed, include the images of the breast biopsy and postbiopsy); (2) pathology slides and reports; (3) results from blood work; and (4) body scans (if applicable). These items can be collected by you for delivery in person or shipped by an overnight carrier, which will track and guarantee delivery. Electronic documents, images, and scans can also be e-mailed directly from you or from your diagnosing doctor's office. In addition, most facilities will give you a health history questionnaire that includes space for you to provide a thorough family history of breast cancer on your mother's and father's sides of the family. (See chapter 13 for a discussion of family history pedigrees.) The second-opinion coordinator will most likely send you this questionnaire, to be completed and returned by mail or in person at the time of the consult.

It is not always necessary to obtain a second opinion in person. Traditionally, patients seeking additional expert advice would schedule an appointment with a local physician or medical center, take along to this appointment the pathology report, biopsy slides, and imaging pictures from their diagnosing doctor, and obtain the second opinion during the consult. Now that most medical records are available electronically and with easy access to overnight shipping, it is possible to receive a second opinion without traveling a great distance for an in-person meeting. If you desire a second opinion from someone whom you consider to be a breast cancer expert, whether that person is in your state, somewhere else in the United States, or even in another country, this can be accomplished. The second opinion can be delivered back to you electronically or by regular mail for you to review and discuss with your treating physician.

Based on your medical records, images, and pathology, the second-opinion specialist(s) will present their assessment of your diagnosis, recommend treatment options, and discuss the risks and benefits of those options. The price you pay for this time and expertise will be money well spent. You should feel confident your diagnosis is correct, and be comfortable with the information you have received. Remember, differences in approach and treatment do occur. What is extremely important in a second opinion is to confirm the cancer diagnosis and the results from the pathology so that you receive the appropriate treatment for your type and extent of cancer. A misdiagnosis in this area can lead to over- or undertreatment; a second opinion can help to reduce this possibility.

For the most part, physicians, like people everywhere, have different ways of approaching a problem and believe that what they are doing is best and have their reasons for their treatment choices. You must consider the opinions presented and choose the treatment plan that is right for you. There is a good chance that the second opinion will simply confirm the diagnosis and treatment suggested by your first doctor.

Armed with your first and second opinions and the reading and research you have done, you are now ready to review all the information with your physician and settle on a comprehensive treatment plan. This may be hard for you to believe, but you can reach this point in a two- to three-week period. While you may think you will never be able to decide on your own treatment, you may be pleasantly surprised. In the upcoming weeks, you will find that your confidence and desire to participate in your own care will increase with the amount of information and guidance you have. It is not a path you would have chosen but one you must take, and the better prepared you are, the safer the journey!

To help you compare the information provided in first and second opinions, we have included the accompanying worksheet (worksheet 2.1).

Working within the Medical System

✖ Medical offices all function and work differently. It would be ideal to have access to every doctor in every office whenever you need them, but this is not always possible. The following are a few key points to help you navigate the different medical systems.

- Carry a notebook or electronic record-keeping tool that is set up to record information received from the different medical offices.
- Have at hand all necessary contact information, including names and telephone numbers.
- Discuss how best to communicate with your medical team: telephone, e-mail, etc.

SECOND OPINION WORKSHEET			
Tumor Characteristics and Opinions			**Notes and Decisions**
	Primary Opinion	Second Opinion	
SIZE			
Palpable			
Mammogram			
Ultrasound			
PATHOLOGY			
Invasive			
Noninvasive			
Histologic grade			
Hormone +/-			
Her2 +/-			
Lymph nodes			
TREATMENT			
Local control			
Systemic control			
FOLLOW-UP			
Hormonal			
Surveillance			
Clinical trials			

Worksheet 2.1

Second opinion worksheet

- Ask about the procedures for urgent assistance. (Your own doctor may not be available, but that is OK. You will speak either to the doctor on call or to other medical personnel responsible for helping you.)
- Inquire at each medical office how you can obtain a copy of your personal records.
- Learn the name and telephone number of the person at every office who is responsible for the business aspects of your treatment, who processes insurance claims, treatment authorizations, requests for medical records, etc.

There is nothing more distressing than being diagnosed with cancer and then having to deal in a new environment that is intimidating and foreign at the same time. Many find this combination simply overwhelming. Your task is further complicated by the fact that you will need to see a number of different physician specialists, requiring you to interact and coordinate several different offices and treatment facilities at the same time.

Every office and treatment facility has key individuals you will get to know. There is usually a clinical person (registered nurse, nurse practitioner, or physician's assistant) who works closely with the physician, and whom you can contact *between office visits* for any questions or concerns. This person has direct access to your doctor and can act as your advocate, especially if he or she knows you and is familiar with your current medical and treatment status. The nurse or nurse practitioner can most likely get to the physician faster than you can, so for this reason we recommend that you utilize this team member as your first choice for help.

To address key specific issues with your doctor, be sure to keep a list of your concerns and questions so that you don't forget anything at your next office visit. In the next section we will discuss the importance of collecting and managing your personal health records.

Your Medical Information and Experiences

Your Medical Records
We believe it is important for all patients to track their personal health information. By keeping up-to-date, easily accessible health records you will play an active role in your breast cancer treatment and become an informed and knowledgeable participant in your care and survival plan.

Maintaining your breast cancer medical records will help you to:

- keep track of every aspect of your care
- provide easy and direct access to your complete breast cancer medical history
- know and understand your personal breast cancer diagnosis and treatment plan
- easily retain and share medical information with healthcare providers
- ensure that all members of your medical team are informed and united on the course of your care
- avoid the possibility of incorrect treatment
- reduce or eliminate the potential for duplicate procedures or tests
- prevent delays in treatment and decision-making

We suggest you adopt an organized approach to collecting your medical information right from the start. You can collect, organize, and store your medical information in a number of different ways:

1. Simply gather your paper records and file them in a three-ring binder using tabs for the various types of documents, for example: physician or medical office contact information, insurance records, office visit notes, pathology reports, surgical procedures, chemotherapy treatment schedule, appointment calendar, and so on.

2. Create a folder in your personal computer and transfer medical records obtained electronically from your health care providers into the dedicated location. You can sort your medical documents into different subfolders within your breast cancer folder, such as those described above.

3. Subscribe to a Web-based electronic tool that allows you to enter and access your health information by computer at any time. Using a Web-based medical records application allows you to receive and store all personal health documents related to your breast cancer diagnosis and treatment, including radiology images, surgical reports, lab results, chemotherapy regimen, appointment calendar, office visit notes, pharmacy and prescription records, and much more.

To help with the process of collecting and storing your personal medical records electronically, we have created a breast cancer specific application that can be accessed at: http://www.drjohnlink. com.

Whichever method you choose will allow you to retain a complete picture of your breast cancer history that you can review at any time and if you choose, to share with family, friends, or other health care providers. Your health information will most likely be scattered across many different medical facilities and provider offices so you will want to establish how these individual sites will provide information to you, whether by paper copy, e-mail, or through another type of electronic transmission such as fax or e-fax. Having direct access to your medical records allows you the opportunity and ability to absorb complex information about your diagnosis, treatment, and test results and to actively participate in your survival.

Record Medical Sessions

At our breast care centers, we routinely record consultations and second opinion sessions. At the conclusion of the appointment a CD copy is made for patients to take home with them. We understand that an extensive amount of information is exchanged that may be new to you or that you might not remember due to feelings of anxiety, stress, or fear. If a member of your personal support team cannot attend the consultation with you, then obtaining a recording of the session will provide you with an accurate accounting to share later. Through review of the recorded session you will have an opportunity to more fully absorb the information presented and many of your questions may be answered. If your breast care facility does not currently utilize a method to record important sessions, our Web-based tool described above contains a helpful link to a site that can assist you with this process.

Keep a Personal Journal

The process of writing down your experiences, thoughts, and feelings can be very beneficial and healing. Researchers at the University of Texas at Austin and North Dakota State University examined healthy people and found that those who write in journals about their deepest thoughts and feelings of difficult events have stronger immunity than those who don't. Another group of researchers from the State University of New York at Stonybrook showed that writing about a stressful experience reduces physical symptoms in patients with chronic illness. Journal writing provides you with the gentlest and safest of therapies. No expertise is required and it is a great way to express yourself without fear of consequence.

Get the Most out of Your Appointments

We want your experience at the doctor's office to be as productive as possible. At your initial appointments, you will be getting details about your breast cancer diagnosis and your treatment options. It's a good idea to bring a list of questions for the doctor. As noted earlier, you might ask if you can record the sessions, if no recordings will be provided. You should consider bringing a loved one or a close friend along with you to help you gather and retain information as well as to provide comfort and reassurance.

The next step is to proceed through the following chapters to ensure that you have a basic knowledge of your breast cancer. By developing a good understanding, you will be sure to ask the questions that are most important in making a truly informed decision. And remember, just take it one step at a time!

3
. . . . . .

Types of Breast Cancer

Over the last several years there has been tremendous scientific interest in understanding the different gene mutations found in breast cancers. As a result, a new classification system for naming breast cancer has emerged. In the past, breast cancer was classified by several different characteristics: (1) the type of cell where the tumor originated (ductal vs. lobular), (2) how different the cancer cell was from the normal breast cell (*differentiation*), and (3) whether the cancer cell contained unique receptors on its surface.

The new classification now being used by research scientists and the medical community was established using a gene analysis technique called *microarray analysis*. In this analysis breast cancer cells are very closely examined (*sequenced*) in the laboratory using special equipment. The results of this analysis have identified *four* distinct breast cancer types.

1. Luminal A
2. Luminal B
3. Basal cell (also called triple-negative)
4. Her2-positive

Each type presents a different pattern of growth, with different ability to spread beyond the breast, and different disease outcome. Establishing your breast cancer type will help guide your medical team to the best treatment options for you.

Until very recently an individual woman's tumor tissue did not routinely undergo microarray analysis as the technique is expensive and was generally used as a research tool. However, specialty laboratories are now beginning to offer commercially available microarray analysis to identify the four different breast cancer types. Even without microarray analysis, your cancer will still be categorized into one of the four types based on the following: (1) the way it looks under the microscope (the unique characteristics of the cancer cell and how much it looks like or differs in appearance from a normal cell), (2) where the cancer began (duct or lobule), (3) the presence or absence of hormone receptors (estrogen and progesterone) on the surface of the cancer cell, and (4) the production of a cancer gene known as the *Her2 oncogene.*

The incidence of each of the four breast cancer types is presented in the accompanying pie graph (Figure 3.1). Your pathology report may not list your type, but this practice is changing and in the future typing information will be included routinely on pathology reports.

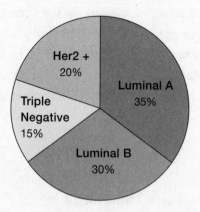

Figure 3.1

Distribution of breast cancer types

Using the descriptions that follow, you can easily determine your type, and your oncologist will certainly work with you to understand which category your tumor falls into. Chapter 7 describes the treatment regimens appropriate for each of these breast cancer types.

1. Luminal A

✺ Luminal A cancers are slow-growing, *low-grade* cancers. They are the breast cancers most frequently discovered by screening mammograms. In the older classification the Luminal A cancers were the well-differentiated (meaning the cancer cells closely resemble normal cells), grade 1 (or low-grade), ductal cancers (originating in the milk duct). These low-grade breast cancers have excellent outcomes, with cure rates in excess of 90 percent. Subtypes of Luminal A cancers include: tubular, papillary, cribriform, mucinous (also known as colloid) cancers; this terminology is used to describe how the cancer cells appear under the microscope. All Luminal A cancers are estrogen- and progesterone-positive, which means that they have both estrogen and progesterone receptors on the cancer cell surface. They are considered low-grade based on their *modified Bloom-Richardson score* (see chapter 4), and they lack the Her2 overproduction.

When specialized testing is conducted on Luminal A cancer cells, they are found to be very similar to a normal breast tissue cell. The more a cancer cell looks like a normal cell, the more it will behave like one. For this reason I believe we must be careful not to overtreat this cancer type. Luminal A cancers tend to develop in a single site in the breast (*unifocal*) and to remain in that place without spreading into the lymph system or bloodstream. These cancers can be cured with limited surgery and radiation and do not require chemotherapy.

One of the current controversies about Luminal A breast cancers is whether this type can further mutate and change its DNA blueprint over time to become a Luminal B cancer; certain scientific evidence suggests that this can occur. Pathologists examining Luminal A tumor

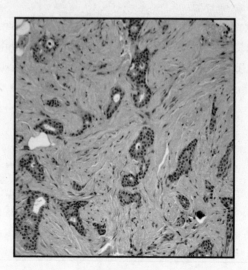

Figure 3.2

Luminal A breast cancer

tissue under the microscope sometimes observe an area within the cancer that appears to be different and has a higher *proliferative rate* (growth rate). If left to continue growing, this mutated group of cells (called a *clone*) can overtake the surrounding slower-growing Luminal A cancer cells. As further evidence, we rarely find a grade 1 cancer larger than 2 centimeters. It is thought that before the Luminal A cancer reaches 2 centimeters it changes into the more aggressive Luminal B type. I believe this is why screening and early diagnosis are so important, in order to find small cancers before they have a chance to change and become more dangerous.

2. Luminal B

✂ In the old classification Luminal B cancers were termed intermediate-grade ductal cancers *or* infiltrating lobular cancers. Sometimes they are a mixture of both ductal and infiltrating lobular cancers which is called *mammary carcinoma*. As stated in the previous section, some Luminal A cancers probably become Luminal B over time. These transformed cancers tend to be more aggressive in their growth and spread than Luminal A. They are estrogen receptor–positive but often lose the progesterone receptor from the cancer cell surface. They do not overproduce the Her2 oncogene. Luminal B cancers have a higher proliferative rate (growth rate) and increased *Ki67 score* (a measure of how quickly cancer cells are growing) than Luminal A cancers.

Those that have a *lobular* pattern are frequently *multifocal* (the cancer develops at multiple sites within one quadrant of the breast), with *skipped* areas of normal breast tissue in between. The mammogram will often underestimate the size of the primary cancer and not identify the secondary *satellite* cancers. For this reason, MRI is often a very helpful imaging tool with Luminal B cancers.

Treatment of Luminal B cancers requires special considerations. Local control requires removing the cancer completely from the breast, and because of the multifocality and difficulty determining the extent of the cancer on physical exam and imaging, complete removal is often challenging. It is not unusual to find cancer at the edge of the removed

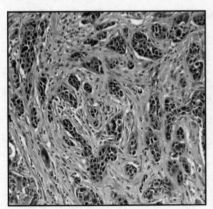

Figure 3.3a

Luminal B: ductal subtype

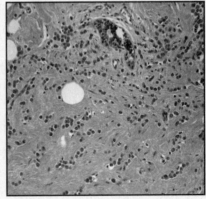

Figure 3.3b

Luminal B: lobular subtype

breast tissue (*positive margins*), making a second surgery necessary to achieve *clear margins*.

Compared with Luminal A cancers, Luminal B cancers have a greater ability or propensity to spread through the lymph and blood vessels. New technologies using *gene profiling* have helped the medical oncologist to determine those women who will benefit from chemotherapy after surgery. (Treatment for Luminal B cancers is discussed further in chapter 6.)

3. Basal Type or Triple-Negative

Basal-type cancers account for about 20 percent of all breast cancer. These cancers are also termed *triple-negative* (the term most frequently used by the medical and patient community) because they often lack both estrogen and progesterone hormone receptors on their cell surfaces and they do not overproduce the Her2 oncogene. Close to 90 percent of basal-type cancers are truly triple-negative. The remaining 10 percent do have some degree of hormone positivity on the cell surface but do not respond to hormone therapy.

Triple-negative cancers are very proliferative, with high Ki67 percentage and high modified Bloom-Richardson scores. In other words, these cancers tend to be fast growing, spreading, and aggressive. Basal-type breast cancers are more prevalent in young women, and they often present as a palpable mass. Ninety percent of breast cancer in women who are carriers for the *BRCA1* gene mutation is the basal type, compared to fourteen percent in *BRCA2* carriers (see chapter 13).

The triple-negative type of breast cancer has received much attention from researchers. Breast cancer cells are most sensitive to chemotherapeutic agents when the cells are actively reproducing and growing. As previously noted, triple-negative cancer cells are highly active, and because of their high proliferation rate they are quite sensitive to chemotherapy. The treatment—as well as prognosis—for triple-

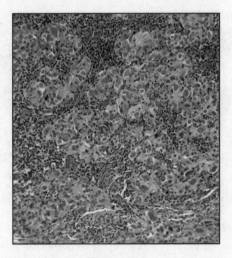

Figure 3.4
Basal type or Triple-negative

negative cancers is evolving with the discovery of new agents and methods to deliver them. (This is further discussed in chapter 6.)

4. Her2-Positive

✂ Approximately 20 percent of breast cancers overproduce a gene called the *Her2 oncogene*. This oncogene (a gene that can cause cancer) promotes the growth of cancer cells by sending messages to the cells to grow and to spread. Cancers that are positive for the Her2 oncogene tend to be more aggressive than other types of breast cancer, and they are either hormone-positive or -negative, which will influence decisions about future hormone treatment. These fast-growing cancers have high Ki67 and high modified Bloom-Richardson scores. Like basal type breast cancer, this type is more prevalent in younger women and is usually found as a rapidly growing breast mass. Diagnosis of Her2-positive breast cancer depends on identifying the presence of *Her2*

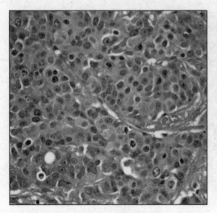

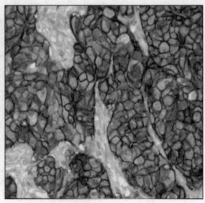

Figure 3.5a
Her2-positive

Figure 3.5b
Her2-positive with IHC staining

receptors on the cell surface using a special *immunohistochemical* (IHC) test, a process that stains the receptors so that they are easier to see under the microscope (Figures 3.5a and 3.5b).

The IHC staining provides a score of 0, 1, 2, or 3 based on the number of Her2 receptors that are seen on the cell surface. Zero and 1 are considered *negative* for Her2 oncogene, while 3 is positive for over-production of Her2. A 2 is *indeterminate* and requires an additional test to measure the Her2 oncogene *inside* the cell using a fluorescent stain known as *fluorescence in situ hybridization* (FISH). A third method that measures gene over-activity, known as *reverse transcription* polymerase chain reaction (RT-PCR) is now commercially available. It is critical to accurately determine if a breast cancer produces the Her2 receptor because a highly effective therapy has been specifically developed to treat this type of cancer. (The therapy is not effective with other breast cancers.)

The tremendous progress made in the treatment of Her2-positive breast cancer is due to our increased understanding of the *molecular pathways* within the cell and the development of chemical agents that can disrupt the pathways. An antibody to the Her2 receptor (Herceptin) when added to chemotherapy has greatly increased the cure rate for Her2-positive breast cancer (chapter 7). Further understanding of the

New Classification	Hormone Receptors: Estrogen (ER) and Progesterone (PR)	Modified Bloom-Richardson Score	Ki-67
Luminal A	Strong for both	low	low
Luminal B	ER is positive, PR is often weak	intermediate	intermediate
Basal type	Negative	high	high
Her2-positive	Positive or negative	high	high

Table 3.1

New Classification of breast cancer

intracellular (inside the cell) pathways has led to the discovery of additional targeted chemical agents (lapatinib, neratinib) that can block signals within the cells, causing the cells to die. To me, this is one of the most exciting areas of breast cancer treatment—understanding the molecular basis of the malignant process that can lead to the development of targeted treatments capable of reversing the process.

The new classification replaces the previous one, which divided breast cancers into two cell types: *invasive ductal carcinoma* and *infiltrating lobular carcinoma*. Ductal cancer can be any of the four cell types, but lobular falls into the Luminal B category. Ductal cancers originate in the duct just before the duct ends in the *lobule*. Lobules are *globes* of glandular cells that produce milk, and it is believed that lobular cancers originated from these cells. As discussed in chapter 1, the beginnings of cancer can remain within the confines of the ductal system—what is termed *in situ*. *Ductal carcinoma in situ* (DCIS) is discussed at length in chapter 5.

Within the lumen of the lobule an in situ lesion can develop that was previously called *lobular carcinoma in situ* (LCIS). Because LCIS actually represents a premalignant condition it is now referred to as *lobular neoplasia*. Unlike DCIS, the cells inside the lobules do not form calcification. We are not even sure that lobular neoplasia leads to invasive breast cancer. This is an area of ongoing discussion and controversy among the medical and research communities. What we do know is that lobular neoplasia is often associated with infiltrating lobular cancer, but it is not clear that it is the precursor. Lobular neoplasia that is discovered as an incidental finding *with or without* an associated cancer increases a woman's risk of developing breast cancer in the future. This cancer can be any of the four previously described types but is most often associated with Luminal B. The finding of lobular neoplasia is very important in treatment planning and future risk reduction strategies.

Rare Breast Cancers

Medullary Breast Cancer

Most often seen in younger women, medullary cancers are dense, cellular, and well circumscribed, meaning they are round with a clearly defined border. Under the microscope this cancer is high-grade and looks menacing, but often has immune response cells surrounding the border. In spite of its appearance under the microscope, medullary cancer has a much better prognosis than a high-grade ductal cancer of equivalent size. However, because this diagnosis is somewhat difficult— due to the close similarity between medullary cancer and high-grade ductal cancer—many pathologists request an outside opinion. When there is doubt or controversy, it is recommended that patients be treated for high-grade ductal cancer, which usually means chemotherapy.

Cystosarcoma Phyllodes

This unusual tumor can be noncancerous or malignant. The distinction can be difficult for the pathologist to make. This cancer's presentation is usually that of an enlarging mass in the breast of a young woman. Clinically and on scans and other imaging, the lump usually looks and feels like a benign tumor known as a *fibroadenoma*, a common occurrence in young women. However, these lesions can grow large and grow rapidly, unlike fibroadenomas, which seldom exceed 2 centimeters. When the healthy cell converts into its malignant form, it resembles a sarcoma; it does not spread to lymph nodes, and it does not involve the duct system. The malignant form rarely spreads into the blood system. The treatment of choice is surgery, and lymph node sampling is not necessary. Patients with large tumors, which make breast conservation impossible without major deformity, should consider a skin-sparing type of mastectomy with immediate reconstruction. In our experience, the nipple and areola can be spared because cystosarcoma phyllodes tumors do not involve the ducts.

Metaplastic Breast Cancer

Under the microscope metaplastic breast cancer has the characteristics of cancer types other than breast cancer. Almost always *triple-negative*, it is aggressive and rapidly divides, requiring adjuvant chemotherapy. At our centers, we send samples of metaplastic breast cancer to laboratories that perform *molecular pathway profiling* in order to help us select the most appropriate chemotherapy.

Paget's Disease

Paget's disease of the breast presents as a scaly, itchy nipple. It is a persistent problem, and often women first seek medical help from a dermatologist. Paget's disease is an in situ breast cancer of the nipple ducts that is frequently associated with underlying invasive breast cancer (approximately 50 percent of the time). This possibility should be carefully investigated. The treatment of choice is a wide excision of the nipple-areolar complex.

Inflammatory Breast Cancer

Inflammatory Breast Cancer (IBC) mimics infection of the breast (*mastitis*) and does not respond to antibiotics. It is an aggressive cancer that is usually triple-negative and spreads rapidly through the lymphatic system under the skin of the breast, resulting in what appears to be a *dermatitis* (inflammation of the skin). Diagnosis is often made by a skin biopsy. The treatment for IBC is chemotherapy followed by surgery (mastectomy) and radiation. This cancer, once almost always fatal, now has a much better prognosis with aggressive systemic chemotherapy given prior to surgery.

Special Types of Luminal A Breast Cancer: Tubular, Papillary, (Mucinous or Colloid), and Cribriform

These variants of Luminal A breast cancer have an excellent prognosis and are treated with surgery. The risk of systemic spread is minimal.

CHECKPOINTS

1. What is my breast cancer type?
2. What is the probability of cure for my type of breast cancer?
3. What are the statistical chances of a local recurrence?
4. What are the statistical chances of a systemic recurrence?

4
. . . . . .
❧

The Pathology Report

You will want to review and understand your pathology report. Historically, physicians often believed that it was better for patients to have limited access to their medical reports. Doctors wanted to interpret the medical jargon prior to presentation to the patient because they were concerned that patients might misunderstand the information contained in the report. This thinking has changed among the medical community today. The philosophy at our breast centers and at many others is that it is important for you to read and understand your pathology report, even if it contains confusing or bad news. We want to help you understand the meaning of this health information so that you can become an integral part of your own health team. Our group has worked closely with breast pathologists to develop and format a report that provides consistent and meaningful information. When we conduct a second opinion, we review a patient's tissue slides and corresponding pathology report, which includes a written description of the tissue received in the laboratory (called a *macroscopic* or *gross* description).

Most women today will have at least two separate pathology reports. The first is usually from the diagnostic needle biopsy of the cancer, and the second is generated from the breast surgery that follows at a later date. If the cancer is not *palpable* (cannot be felt), the needle biopsy will be obtained using image guidance such as ultrasound, stereotactic, or MRI. Information collected from imaging coupled with the biopsy results will give the treating team important information about planning further treatment.

Historically, the pathology report was a written description of what the pathologist observed when looking at the cancer tissue under the microscope. Usually this was the surgical biopsy tissue from a mastectomy or partial mastectomy. The pathologist described the nature of the cancer cells or how similar or dissimilar they were from a normal cell (*their degree of differentiation*), the total size of the cancer, whether there appeared to be invasion into the surrounding blood vessels or lymph system, and if there appeared to be any reaction or response to the cancer by the patient's own defense system (*host response*). Usually included along with the surgical specimen were the regional lymph nodes, and the pathologist carefully examined slices of each node to determine if there was cancer spread. From this information the cancer was staged (Stage I, II, or III *or* TNM staging), and it was decided whether radiation was needed. When chemotherapy became available in the late 1970s, information from the pathologic review was critical to ascertain the need for its use. Because of limited options in the early era of breast cancer treatment, the pathologic description of the breast tissue was primarily evaluated to predict patient outcome (*prognosis*). As more sophisticated and innovative therapies and technologies were developed, the pathologic analysis evolved into a health management tool that was able to drive the decision-making around treatment options that would influence a woman's chance for a cure.

While the early analyses presented information that to this day is the bedrock of the pathology report, new developments added to and enhanced our knowledge of the unique aspects of the cancer cell to help us understand the individual patient's cancer characteristics. One major development was the discovery of specialized receptors on the cancer cell surface that soon became targets for therapy. Techniques were developed using special stains that identified the presence or absence of *hormone receptors* on the cancer cell surface. These first *immunohistochemical stains* (IHC) were designed to identify estrogen and progesterone receptors. The presence or absence of the receptors predicted whether hormonal therapies would be effective in controlling the cancer. Indeed, clinical trials did prove that hormonal agents such as tamoxifen and the aromatase inhibitors could effectively kill this type of cancer cell (see chapter 8) in women whose cancer tested positive for hormone receptors.

Much later another type of receptor was found in an especially aggressive breast cancer. Originally called the *epidermal growth factor receptor*, this receptor is now known as the *Her2 receptor*. This development led to the discovery of an important therapeutic drug known as Herceptin that is specifically directed at this receptor. Testing for Her2 receptors, and most likely others in the future, is now an extremely important part of the information contained within the pathology report, and the results are absolutely critical for use in the modern treatment of breast cancer.

Most recently we have entered a new era of *genomic analysis* of cancer cells. Results from this testing are rapidly being incorporated into treatment planning. Investigators are now able to examine genetic differences among cancers and identify genes that are associated with invasion, spread, aggressiveness, and metastasis. We are in the early days of these types of analyses, but we can already examine tumor tissue to identify women who are likely to relapse and who will therefore benefit from chemotherapy. Equally important, genetic analysis of this type identifies women who will *not* benefit from chemotherapy, thus preventing unnecessary treatment with the associated side effects. Because we have only just entered the realm of genomic analysis, the highly specialized testing is performed in a limited number of laboratories.

Today's pathology report still contains the physical description of the cancer and the measurement of its size. Based on new and innovative research developments, the pathology report also states whether cell surface receptors are present or absent and often provides the results of genomic analysis. In the future we can expect that the pathology report will include all of this and more. We cannot emphasize enough that accurate and thorough pathology reporting is critical to predicting outcome and prognosis. Planning appropriate treatment based on the pathology report will result in increased patient survival.

Now that we have discussed the important role that the pathology report plays in your diagnosis and treatment, I want to help you to read and understand your own pathology report.

Pathology Report: Needle Biopsy

✂ Ninety percent of newly diagnosed women will receive a breast cancer diagnosis based on a needle biopsy resulting from detection of a palpable breast lump or from an abnormality identified by mammogram. The biopsy is a small cylinder of tissue the diameter of a pencil lead and about 5 millimeters long. Even though it is very small, the pathologist is able to obtain a tremendous amount of information about the cancer from the needle biopsy, and this information is formally presented on the pathology report (see Figure 4.1. Sample pathology report from needle biopsy). The report may differ somewhat from laboratory to laboratory; however, the information presented is fairly standard across institutions and will most likely contain the following sections:

Patient identifying information
Final diagnosis
Microscopic description
Molecular studies
Clinical and gross description
Pathologist signature and date of review
Signature of confirming pathologist review

The pathologist will observe the tissue under the microscope and determine if the cancer is confined to the ducts (DCIS) or if it has

Hill Crest Hospital   (999)999-9999   George C. Scott, M.D., Lab Director
Patient name: Maxine Libby
MR# AB12345678   DOB: 01/01/1956

Specimen #: P-7777-23   Date collected: 06/09/2011   Received in lab: 06/09/2011
Specimen type: BREAST BIOPSY, NEEDLE

Final Diagnosis
(Microscopic)

Right Breast, Core Biopsy: —Infiltrating Ductal Carcinoma, High Grade

Summary for invasive breast carcinoma in core biopsy

Anatomic location: Right Breast (12:00)

Needle Biopsy Guidance: Core Biopsy, (NOS)

Result for Surgery: Irregular Mass

Imaging Size of lesion: 1.8 cm
                          (Pathologic tumor size deferred to excisional specimens)

Histologic Type: Infiltrating ductal carcinoma

Tumor Grade: SBR 8/9 (high)
                -Tubules: 3/3
                -Nuclear grade: 3/3
                -Mitosis: 2/3

Prognostic Markers: Performed

Ductal Carcinoma in Situ: Not present

Microcalcifications: Not identified

Lymphatic invasion: Absent

Molecular Studies
Breast Cancer Prognostic Markers

Specimen: Formalin fixed, paraffin block 0

Procedure: Immunohistochemistry, LSAB detection method

Assay: Estrogen Receptors
        Results: Negative   Favorable result: Positive 1–3+

Assay: Progesterone Receptors
        Results: Negative   Favorable result: Positive 1–3+

Assay: Her2/neu
        Results: Negative, 1+   Favorable result: Negative 0–1+

Clinical
Pre-op diagnosis: Right breast, 12 o'clock, irregular mass 1.8 cm

Post-op diagnosis: Suspect malignant

Gross Description:

Labeled right breast is a 1.2 x 0.5 x 0.2 cm aggregate of yellow-tan fibrofatty tissue.
Formalin fixation time, 9 hours.

Signed: Dr. Steven R. Johnson   **Date:** 06/10/11

Findings reviewed and confirmed by: Dr. Frank Wong **Date:** 06/11/11

Figure 4.1

Sample pathology report from needle biopsy

invaded through the basement membrane of the ducts into the surrounding tissue to become an invasive (or infiltrating) breast cancer.

If the pathologist interprets the biopsy as entirely ductal carcinoma in situ (DCIS), the report will be moderately different than if there is invasion present. DCIS and its pathologic characteristics and treatments are thoroughly discussed in chapter 5. The focus of this chapter will be the pathology report for an invasive breast cancer. If the breast cancer has been found to be invasive, the pathologist will determine the grade of the cancer. *Grade* is defined as the degree of malignancy— how far the cells have changed from the original normal cell (or the cell of origin). The pathologist uses a scaling system called the *modified Bloom-Richardson Scale* (MBR) to determine the grade. Three separate characteristics of the cancer cells will be examined: (1) the amount of tubule formation, (2) the nuclear size, and (3) the number of cells in active cell division (*mitosis*). The MBR system assigns a score of 1–3 for *each* characteristic, with 1 being least, or smallest, and 3 being most, or largest. A minimum score of 3 and a maximum score of 9 can be achieved with this system. In Table 4.1 this cancer is given a 2 for tubule formation, a 2 for nuclear size, and a 1 for mitotic rate. This results in a total score of 5 out of a possible 9, written as 5/9. This score is consistent with a Luminal A breast cancer as depicted in Figure 3.2 in chapter 3.

Scores of 3, 4, or 5 are considered low-grade, 6 or 7 are intermediate

Tumor cell characteristics	1	2	3
Tubule formation		X	
Nuclear size		X	
Mitotic rate	X		

Table 4.1

Determining total MBR score

Grade	MBR Score
Low (1)	3, 4, 5
Intermediate (2)	6, 7
High (3)	8, 9

Table 4.2

Determining tumor grade using the MBR score

grade, and 8 or 9 are high-grade cancers (Table 4.2). As described in the previous example, an MBR score of 5 is consistent with a low-grade (1) breast cancer.

The next task for the pathologist is to describe the cancer cells and their patterns as seen under the microscope. Pathologists traditionally have segregated breast cancers into ductal versus lobular patterns. This distinction is still important because lobular cancers have unique characteristics. They tend to be larger than they appear on the breast images, they tend to have satellite foci (which may appear as individual specks), and they are often associated with an increased incidence of a second cancer in the future. Lobular cancers fall into the Luminal B group in the new classification (chapter 3). Under the microscope they do not form tubules, and they appear to branch or "flow" into the fat and supporting tissue in the surrounding breast. Lobular cancers are hormone-positive and Her2-negative almost without exception. A special stain called *e-cahedrin* when applied to the biopsy tissue can help the pathologist distinguish between ductal and lobular carcinomas.

The pathologist will sometimes describe special patterns of growth or arrangement of the cancer cells such as *papillary* or *cribriform* or *tubular*, which are, I believe, somewhat outdated terms having little relevance today. These three tend to be subsets of low-grade ductal cancers (chapter 5). More important is the description of whether the

cancer cells have invaded the lymph or vascular structures, information that is associated with increased spread to the lymph nodes and
which has important treatment implications.

Next the pathologist can perform tests in which different stains are
put on thin slices of the needle biopsy, and which give the treating team
useful information for making treatment decisions. This technique,
called *immunohistochemical staining* (IHC), is able to detect the presence
of specific proteins within the cell and on the cell surface. The four
most common IHC tests identify: (1) estrogen receptors, (2) progesterone receptors, (3) Her2, or (4) Ki67. The hormone receptors and Her2
receptor tests aid in the selection of targeted treatment options and help
to determine the cancer type. The Ki67 test identifies cancer cells that
are preparing to divide. The percentage of cells that are positive for
Ki67 determines how rapidly the cancer is growing (proliferation rate).
In other words, a high Ki67 score indicates a fast growing cancer.

Results from the pathologist review are so critically important to
the decision-making and treatment-planning that most laboratories
require an independent second review to confirm the diagnosis of
cancer. The important information obtained from the biopsy, combined with that from imaging and the clinical exam, provides the
framework for treatment planning. Even more information about the
cancer can be obtained by sending a portion of the biopsy to specialized laboratories for further gene analysis. This testing identifies
whether genes within the cell involved in cell proliferation, invasion,
and metabolic spread are active. Presently, two commercial companies
are performing this gene testing in breast cancer. Agendia performs a
seventy-gene analysis, or assay, that is called MammaPrint. The second company, Genomic Health, performs a twenty-one-gene assay
called Oncotype DX. Both of these tests are used in Luminal cancers
to determine increased risk of systemic spread and the need for chemotherapy. I suspect that more of these gene tests will become available in the near future as our knowledge of the malignant process
expands. Not only will these tests predict the risk of systemic spread,
but they will identify which targeted drugs should be used.

Pathology Report: Surgical

❧ The second pathology report occurs following the surgical removal of the cancer. This surgery may be a *wide local excision (WLE)*, also known as a *lumpectomy*, or it may be a mastectomy. Often the surgery involves removal of one or more lymph nodes (see chapter 6). A course of preoperative (*neoadjuvant*) chemotherapy may occur *before* either of these surgeries, which can greatly alter the extent and appearance of the cancer. It is not uncommon for there to be *no cancer remaining* at the time of surgery, which is called a *complete pathologic response*.

The surgical pathology report describes the size of the invasive cancer and the associated in situ cancer, if any. It notes the presence or absence of lymph node involvement, and provides details on the cancer cells' appearance under the microscope, along with MBR grade. If IHC stains were not performed on the needle biopsy, they can be performed now for estrogen and progesterone receptors, Her2 receptors, and Ki67. The surgical pathology report may include information from the prior needle biopsy. (Figure 4.2 provides a sample surgical pathology report.)

The goal of surgery is to remove the cancer completely plus a rim of normal tissue around it. When the surgeon removes the cancer he orients it for the pathologist using small clips. The pathologist examines the removed specimen under the microscope and determines if there is clearance of normal tissue completely surrounding the cancer (clear margins) and to what extent (measurement in mm). This information is presented on the pathology report under *Margins of resection*.

Included in the surgical pathology report is the stage of the breast cancer. The staging system involves the extent of the primary cancer and the spread to the lymph nodes. This system is called the *TNM system*, where *T* is tumor size, *N* is number of lymph nodes, and M is metastatic disease (spread to another part of the body). (Figure 4.3 describes the TNM strategy.)

Historically, the TNM staging system was correlated to prognosis and survival, but today I believe it has less relevance. This system does

Hill Crest Hospital (999)999-9999 George C. Scott, M.D., Lab Director Page 1 of 2
Patient name: Maxine Libby
MR# AB12345678 DOB: 01/01/1956

Specimen #: P-7777-23 Date collected: 06/09/2011 Received in lab: 06/09/2011
Specimen type: Partial mastectomy

Final Diagnosis
(Microscopic)

Right Breast, Partial mastectomy: Infiltrating Ductal Carcinoma, High Grade
Summary for invasive breast carcinoma in partial mastectomy
Anatomic location: Right Breast (12:00)
Size of specimen: 6 x 5 x 5 cm
Size of tumor: 1.8 cm
Histologic Type: Infiltrating ductal carcinoma, High grade
Tumor Grade: MBR 8/9 (high)
-Tubules: 3/3
-Nuclear grade: 3/3
-Mitosis: 2/3
Tumor necrosis: Not present
Margins of resection: Free of tumor
Prognostic Markers: Performed
Stage: $T_{1c}N_{1a}$
Nipple involvement: NA
Ductal Carcinoma in Situ: Not present
Microcalcifications: None
Lymph nodes: 1/11 nodes positive for cancer

Molecular Studies
Breast Cancer Prognostic Markers
Specimen: Formalin fixed, paraffin block 0
Procedure: Immunohistochemistry, LSAB detection method
Assay: Estrogen Receptors
Results: Negative Favorable result: Positive 1–3+
Assay: Progesterone Receptors
Results: Negative Favorable result: Positive 1–3+
Assay: Her2/neu
Results: Negative, 1+ Favorable result: Negative 0–1+

Clinical
Pre-op diagnosis: Right breast cancer
Specimen(s)
A. Right breast tissue
B. Right axillary contents
Gross Description:
A. Is received fresh, labeled "right breast mass" fatty tissue measuring 6 x 5 x 5 cm.

Signed: Dr. Steven R. Johnson **Date:** 06/10/11
Findings reviewed and confirmed by: Dr. Frank Wong **Date:** 06/11/11

Figure 4.2

Sample surgical pathology report

Tumor size	
T_0	In situ (with no invasion)
T_{1a}, T_{1b}, or T_{1c}	1a: 0–5 mm, 1b: 5–10 mm, 1c: 10–20 mm
T_2	20–50 mm
T_3	>50 mm
T_4	Invasion into the skin or underlying muscle
Lymph node involvement	
N_0	No node involvement
N_{1a}	1–3 nodes involved
N_{1b}	4–10 nodes involved
N_{1c}	>10 nodes involved
Distant spread	
M_x	Unknown if cancer spread to distant site
M_0	No spread to distant site
M_+	Cancer spread to a distant site

Table 4.3

TNM staging

not take into consideration the biology or aggressiveness of the cancer, which is more important in prognosis than the extent of disease. Women who receive preoperative chemotherapy will never have an accurate pathologic staging of their cancer because treatment will alter what the pathologist will ultimately see under the microscope.

CHECKPOINTS

1. How do I obtain my pathology report? (The hospital pathology department or cancer surgeon?)
2. Is my pathology report formatted so that I can interpret the information for decision-making? If not, will my doctor be available to sit down and explain its contents thoroughly to me?
3. What is the stage of my cancer, using the TNM system?
4. From my pathology report can I determine my type of breast cancer based on the new classification of breast cancer as described in chapter 3?

Ductal Carcinoma in Situ (DCIS)

This chapter is written specifically for women with ductal cancer in situ (DCIS). If you have invasive breast cancer, you will probably want to skip this chapter for now and move on to chapter 6. Because of the increasing incidence of DCIS, about 20 percent of newly diagnosed breast cancer, and the controversies and complexities in management, it is necessary to devote an entire chapter to this topic. More cases of DCIS have been identified in recent years through the increased use of screening mammography. Once it was discovered that clusters of unique calcifications in the breast represented preinvasive nonpalpable cancer, we could diagnose cancer from a mammogram before it went on to become invasive.

The good news with this early form of breast cancer is that it is completely curable with local control because it has not had a chance to spread to lymph and blood vessels. The challenge has been the development of appropriate treatment options to achieve local control. Early attempts at surgeries that were less than mastectomy often failed when the surgical margins were inadequate, leaving microscopic residual cancer behind. To counter this, radiation therapy was added and did seem to increase the local control rate; however, the effects of radiation on tissues made breast reconstruction much more difficult if there was a recurrence requiring mastectomy. Our past experience in treating DCIS indicates that breast conservation is feasible and acceptable when the cancer is small and the surgical margins around the cancer are large. For larger DCIS, mastectomy has become much more accepted as the treatment of choice due to the excellent advances in breast reconstruction. For those DCIS that fall in between lumpectomy (WLE) and mastectomy, radiation is often considered and becomes a major decision to be made by the woman in consultation with her treating doctor. To help with the assessment of a local recurrence risk based on the extent and type of DCIS, prognostic criteria have been created (discussed later in this chapter). It must be remembered that this early cancer can be 100 percent cured with a simple mastectomy and that anything less than this leaves a small risk of recurrence. This is the dilemma that the patient with DCIS and her breast surgeon must discuss.

As discussed in chapter 1, DCIS is a ductal cancer that has not penetrated the basement membrane separating the milk duct from the underlying breast tissue that contains blood and lymph vessels (see Figure 1.2 in chapter 1). If the cancer is found at this stage, there is no risk of its spreading into the blood or lymphatic system, and the risk of dying from breast cancer is essentially zero. Fortunately, DCIS is relatively easy to detect before invasion occurs. On the mammogram DCIS appears as a speckling of calcifications or as a change in the breast structure that has a very characteristic appearance to the radiologist (Figure 5.1). The calcifications are dead cancer cells that have petrified (*calcified*) inside the ducts. These *flecks* of calcium have nothing to do with dietary calcium intake.

Like invasive breast cancer, DCIS is a *heterogeneous* disease. According to the medical literature, a majority of these cancers will become invasive if left untreated or undiscovered. The cell that becomes cancerous can vary in aggressiveness and growth rate. Some forms of DCIS are low grade and very slow growing. Under the microscope, the cells are fairly small and resemble small normal breast ductal cells. This form of DCIS is often associated with calcifications that have a powdery

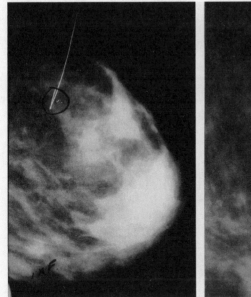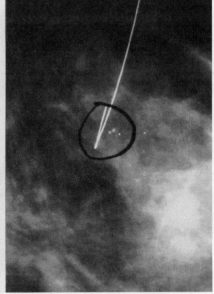

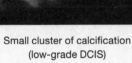

Small cluster of calcification   Magnified view with hook and wire
(low-grade DCIS)

Figure 5.1
Mammogram with calcifications

appearance on the mammogram. Under the microscope, there is little evidence of *necrosis* (dead cellular material) in the center of the ducts (Figure 5.2). Because of the absence of *necrotic* material, known as *comedo necrosis*, this type of DCIS is termed *noncomedo*.

At the other end of the DCIS spectrum is the high-grade form, which is fast growing with many cells dividing. Cancer cells in the center of the duct die, resulting in prominent areas of *central duct necrosis*, and calcifications that look like branching tree limbs (Figure 5.3). If this type of DCIS, termed *comedo*, is allowed to grow and become invasive, it is potentially very dangerous because of its rapid growth rate.

There are also intermediate forms of DCIS that fall between the two ends of the spectrum.

The challenge in treating DCIS is to remove the cancer completely

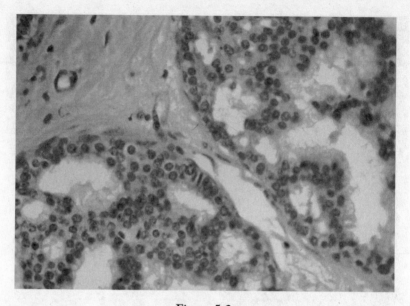

Figure 5.2
Small cell without necrosis

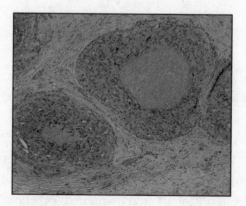

Figure 5.3
DCIS high grade comedo type

from the breast. Surgical excision of the DCIS, along with a clear surrounding *margin* of normal breast tissue, is the primary treatment. The
margin of uninvolved breast tissue is important in preventing a recurrence from cancer cells that could be left behind following surgery.

Ideally, the breast surgeon attempts to remove tissue and leave a 10 millimeter *clear margin* (normal tissue) with normal ducts between the edge of the biopsy and the cancerous duct. This can be difficult if the area of DCIS involvement is large or is close to the skin or chest wall. The extra 10 millimeter margin that the surgeon must remove in these cases can substantially increase the size of the tissue removed and leave the patient with a large deformity or a much smaller breast.

The radiologist can greatly assist the surgeon in planning the best surgical approach possible. Advances in breast MRI have been very helpful to the surgeon, particularly for locating high-grade DCIS. In most cases there is no palpable lump with DCIS; therefore the radiologist must assist the surgeon by placing markers, usually in the form of multiple wire hooks, where the cancer appears in the breast tissue. This guides the surgeon in the operating room to know exactly what portion of breast tissue must be removed.

Breast surgeons learned from early experience that if the area of DCIS was small and they cleared wide margins with an *excisional biopsy*, the cancer would not recur in most women. For larger areas of involvement, it was often impossible for surgeons to clear the margins adequately to prevent recurrence yet leave the breast with an acceptable size and symmetry. In these latter cases, most women chose simple mastectomy, often with immediate reconstruction, resulting in a cure rate of close to 100 percent.

Clinical trials have demonstrated that radiation in addition to surgery reduces the recurrence rates when the cancer's involvement is large and the margins are close. Radiation, however, is less effective when DCIS is high-grade and large with close margins. Additional clinical trials have revealed that the drug tamoxifen (chapter 8) further reduces recurrence rates and also prevents the development of new cancers in the opposite breast. This drug is only effective in patients whose DCIS is *estrogen receptor–positive* (chapter 4).

There are two fundamental treatment decisions to be made in the management of ductal carcinoma in situ. First, is mastectomy required, or can an acceptable local control rate be achieved with less than mastectomy (WLE) and with an acceptable cosmetic result? Second, if a wide local excision (WLE) is possible, should radiation be added to increase the local control rate?

We know that mastectomy provides a 100 percent local control rate and that WLE with or without radiation yields results between 85 and 90 percent. If a recurrence is discovered early, the recurring cancer is usually still DCIS and not life-threatening. Recurrence most often requires mastectomy, and if the patient has received radiation, reconstruction may be more difficult because of radiation effects on tissue elasticity and healing.

To help patients and their surgeons with these decisions physicians at the Van Nuys Breast Center in Southern California and the University of Southern California have developed a system for assessing DCIS and its associated treatment options. The Van Nuys group identified four critical factors that influence local recurrence: (1) the size of the DCIS tumor, (2) the cell type and presence of necrosis, (3) the amount of clear margin, and (4) the age of the patient. Like the modified Bloom-Richardson score (chapter 4) for invasive cancer, each category is given a score of 1, 2, or 3. The scoring grid appears in Table 5.1.

From careful long-term follow-up, the Van Nuys group correlated recurrence rates to the total score. Based on their work and a local

Index	1	2	3
Size	0–14 mm	15–40 mm	>40 mm
Cell type and necrosis	Low and intermediate nuclear grade without necrosis	Intermediate nuclear grade with necrosis	High nuclear grade with necrosis
Extent of clear margin	>10 mm	1–9 mm	<1 mm
Age	>60	40–60	<40

Table 5.1

Van Nuys Prognostic Index (VNPI)

VNPI Score	Treatment recommendation
4, 5, 6	WLE excision
7, 8, 9	WLE + radiation
10, 11, 12	Mastectomy

Table 5.2

Treatment recommendations based on the VNPI score

control rate of greater than 85 percent, the following treatment recommendations are suggested in Table 5.2.

Occasionally, DCIS is discovered just as the cancer has developed the ability to penetrate the basement membrane. This very early invasion (often called *microinvasion*) is reported by the pathologist. When we see microinvasion, we consider it the same as pure DCIS as long as the amount of invasion is small. Once the invasion involves several millimeters, we consider it a small invasive breast cancer.

There is one exception to the above, and it involves a larger DCIS lesion with microinvasion that overexpresses the Her2 oncogene. This rare presentation of DCIS is composed of high-grade cells with prominent central duct necrosis and has multiple areas of microinvasion. This cancer has a small risk of systemic spread (as high as 10 percent), and Herceptin-based systemic therapy should be considered (chapter 7).

Table 5.3 demonstrates the decision flowchart for DCIS. It includes the Van Nuys Prognostic Index scores (VNPI). As can be seen from the flowchart, Decision 1 regards the extent of surgery needed. If wide local excision (WLE) is the decision, the goal is complete removal of the DCIS with greater than 10 millimeter margins. Breast surgeons are becoming more successful in this through the use of innovative *oncoplastic* techniques, moving or relocating breast tissue to replace removed tissue and adjusting the opposite breast to create symmetry and balance. Although the trend has been to add radiation (Decision 2), many women are now choosing simple mastectomy with a planned skin- and sometimes nipple-sparing procedure, which provides close

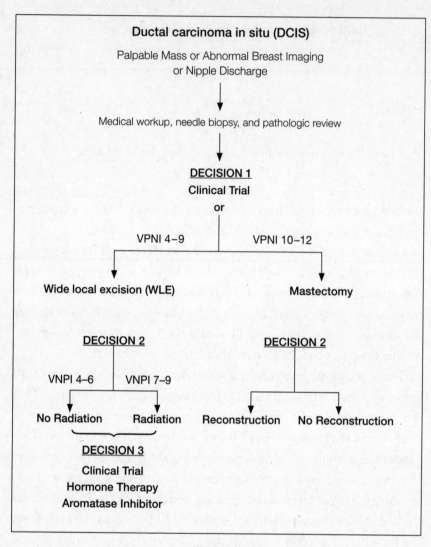

Table 5.3

Decision tree for DCIS, including VNPI

to a 100 percent cure. The nipple can be spared if the DCIS is significantly away from the nipple-areolar complex and a sampling at the time of surgery reveals no nipple involvement.

In summary, DCIS is a relatively newly recognized breast cancer with the advent of screening mammography. It is a breast cancer that is discovered before invasion has occurred. Management is evolving and is at times complicated and should be individualized based on each woman's particular set of circumstances.

CHECKPOINTS

1. Is my surgeon working closely with the radiologist in planning the best surgical procedure to remove the DCIS with adequate margins? Do I need a breast MRI?
2. Is the pathologist reporting the type of DCIS, the presence or absence of necrosis, and a measurement of the cancer-free margin?
3. What is my Van Nuys Prognostic Index Score?
4. What will be the benefit of adding radiation? Will radiation improve local control?
5. What is the benefit of adding tamoxifen? Has the DCIS been tested for estrogen receptors?

6

❦

Invasive Breast Cancer

LOCAL AND SYSTEMIC CONTROL

The cure of breast cancer depends on local control, and if cancer cells have escaped into the bloodstream, it will also depend on systemic control. *Local control* is defined as the complete removal or eradication of the primary cancer in the breast and any disease in adjacent lymph nodes. *Systemic control* is defined as the eradication of any cancer cells that have spread from the original breast cancer through the bloodstream into the rest of the body.

In the previous chapter we discussed ductal carcinoma in situ (DCIS), which accounts for 20 percent of newly diagnosed breast cancer. Now we will address the management of invasive breast cancer, which accounts for the remaining 80 percent. Invasive cancer, as described in chapter 1, is more complicated because of the risk of systemic spread. The four types of invasive breast cancer (defined in chapter 3) have different genomic patterns and vary in clinical presentation, appearance under the microscope, and risk of spread. The cure for invasive breast cancer, regardless of the type, requires local control, and if cancer cells have spread into the body, systemic control will also be needed. Historically, the sequence of treatment was local control first, either surgery or surgery and radiation, followed by systemic therapy: chemotherapy and/or hormonal therapy depending on the risk of spread. Under the old system, staging of the lymph nodes was necessary to determine if systemic therapy was required. Systemic treatment after surgery is called *adjuvant therapy* (added onto surgery).

As discussed in chapter 1, new technology applied to the needle biopsy prior to surgery allows us to assess the risk of systemic spread. With this information we sometimes make the decision to administer systemic treatment prior to surgery. This approach is termed *neoadjuvant* (preoperative) chemotherapy. In appropriate cases there are major benefits in administering systemic therapy prior to surgery, which will be discussed later in this chapter. First, however, we will discuss local control—surgery and radiation. If you are like most women in the crisis of newly diagnosed breast cancer, the most immediate and pressing issue is the removal of the cancer from your breast. A majority of women today still receive local control prior to any consideration of systemic treatment. This is because a majority of newly diagnosed cancers are found early on screening mammograms and are Luminal A or small Luminal B cancers.

Local Control

The objective of local control is to remove the cancer in its entirety. Fifty years ago the only approach was to remove the entire breast—a mastectomy. As screening mammography discovered smaller cancers, clinical trials conducted in the 1970s and '80s demonstrated that local control could be achieved with less surgery—surgery that is called either a *lumpectomy*, or *partial mastectomy*, or *wide local excision* (WLE). We will use the latter term throughout the rest of this manual.

Two major research trials, one in Italy and the other in the United States, proved that WLE plus radiation for smaller cancers gave equal local control rates when compared to mastectomy. Women treated with WLE without radiation had an approximately 30 percent local recurrence rate. These patients with recurrences required a mastectomy;

however, there was *no decrease* in the cure rate. (We will discuss radiation therapy added to WLE in chapter 10.)

At the time of mastectomy or WLE, the regional lymph nodes in the axilla were removed. Figure 1.5 in chapter 1 demonstrates the breast and lymph node drainage. It was thought that local control required removal of a majority of the lymph nodes located in the axilla of the involved breast. This standard lymph node procedure removed the first two levels of nodes—approximately ten to twenty in number. Many women were found to have no cancer cells in the removed nodes, and approximately 10 percent of patients developed permanent swelling of their arm (*lymphedema*). It was discovered that the removal of the nodes at the time of initial surgery did not increase the cure rate, but the presence of cancer cells in one or more nodes predicted an increase in systemic spread and was important in selecting women who would benefit from systemic therapy.

The next important advance was the discovery that breast cancer first spreads to a single node, called the *sentinel lymph node,* before continuing into adjacent nodes in the region. The sentinel lymph node can be easily identified by injecting a special dye and/or radioactive tracer into or around the cancer prior to the surgery. The surgeon is then able to isolate the location of the sentinel node using a radioactivity-sensing probe and with a small incision; the sentinel node is identified by its "blue" color. This procedure is performed when there are no obvious abnormal lymph nodes on physical examination or ultrasound imaging. The node can then be removed at the time of the WLE or mastectomy for analysis, and if no cancer cells are present, no further lymph node removal is necessary. The incidence of lymphedema has dramatically decreased due to the reduction in lymph node removal.

More recent clinical trials have demonstrated that even with a positive sentinel lymph node, extensive removal of additional nodes is not necessary. Since one of the criteria for systemic therapy is the spread to the sentinel lymph node, a positive lymph node will initiate systemic therapy. Recent studies indicate that systemic therapy treats the remaining axillary lymph nodes as well as the rest of the body, and the incidence of local recurrence in the axilla is the same as that following surgical removal of the remaining lymph nodes.

The past fifty years of clinical research studies in breast cancer local control form the basis for our present treatment decisions and can be summarized as follows:

- WLE with radiation is equal to mastectomy for local control in women with T1 and T2 breast cancers (cancers less than 5 cm, see chapter 4).
- Radiation reduces the risk of local recurrence but does not increase cure rate.
- In patients with no obvious abnormal lymph nodes, removal of an uninvolved sentinel lymph node predicts that there is no spread of cancer to the remaining axillary lymph nodes.
- Women with larger cancers (greater than 5 cm) are not good candidates for WLE and require mastectomy.
- Women with larger cancers and positive involvement of the axillary lymph nodes may be candidates for preoperative systemic therapy to shrink the cancer and make WLE a potential local control option.

Because of this progress, the number of women receiving mastectomy and extensive lymph node removal has been greatly reduced. The number of patients cured of breast cancer in the past thirty years has greatly increased, but it has little to do with the extent of the surgery. Local control is necessary and very important, but with good preoperative planning, less surgery is needed. The increase in cure rate is largely due to earlier diagnosis (resulting from earlier detection) and more effective systemic control (discussed later in this chapter).

I should mention that in spite of this progress, over the past several years there has been an increase in the mastectomy rate—particularly among women opting for *bilateral mastectomy* (removal of both breasts). I believe the reasons for this increase are the following:

- Tremendous progress has been made in the area of reconstructive surgery with excellent cosmetic results (see chapter 11).
- Women choosing mastectomy can avoid radiation and greatly reduce future risk of another breast cancer.

With this progress from a single treatment in the past—the mastectomy—the choices have become much more complex. You have time to consider your options and what is optimal for your individual situation. Here are some questions for you to consider with your treatment team.

1. Am I a candidate for limited surgery (WLE)?
2. Am I a candidate for sentinel lymph node removal?
3. Will I need radiation? If so, what are my options for radiation? (See chapter 9.)
4. Would I benefit from systemic therapy prior to surgery?
5. Should I consider mastectomy(ies) and immediate reconstruction? If so, am I a candidate for skin-sparing or even nipple-sparing reconstruction?

Systemic Spread and Control

✺ With local control alone, the majority of women with invasive breast cancer will be cured. However, a minority of women who appear to be cured as a result of local control will ultimately relapse due to systemic spread. This is because microscopic cancer cells escape prior to initiation of local control and, in most cases, end up forming *microdeposits* in bone, lung, and/or liver tissue. Unfortunately, at this time we do not have a completely reliable and accurate test to predict this occurrence. Some progress has been made using antibody-labeled stains that are able to identify breast cancer cells in the bone marrow. Although very promising work is being done in this area, no commercial application of this technology is available—*yet*. Other researchers have developed a test that will screen for the presence of circulating cancer cells in the bloodstream. This technology is able to detect one abnormal cell in one million blood cells. The current problem with both of these tests is the unacceptably high incidence of false negatives, meaning that the majority of patients with *micrometastases* will have a negative test result. Research continues in this important area. If we had an accurate predictive test, we could treat only those women who need therapy for systemic spread and spare those who do not.

Women often ask if they can forgo systemic therapy and receive systemic therapy only if they relapse. Once a woman relapses, she can be treated; unfortunately, the chance of long-term survival and cure is small. If metastatic deposits have become established and are large enough to be found by symptoms or imaging, they can be treated using current agents and they will often regress and disappear, only to return later. At this point the metastatic lesions are usually resistant to the agents that were previously effective.

The chance of completely eradicating metastatic deposits is greatly increased when the tumor burden is minimal and microscopic. As we develop more effective and targeted agents, more women will be cured. We are beginning to see this in Her2-positive metastatic disease, as a small number of women appear to be cured after metastatic relapse when treated with Her2-directed therapy.

For now, our best chance of curing women with microscopic meta-static disease is to treat with chemotherapy and/or hormonal therapy at the time of diagnosis—either before or after surgery. Our task is to select women at increased risk for relapse who need the treatment and avoid treating those who don't.

Historically, predictors of systemic relapse were identified as: (1) tumor size, (2) lymph node involvement, and (3) tumor grade using the modified Bloom-Richardson scoring system. We call these *first-generation prognostic factors*. These were the main factors on which an oncologist based his or her decision whether or not to prescribe adjuvant therapy. With new technology using specialized antibody stains (IHC), second generation prognostic factors were identified that not only increased our ability to predict recurrence but they also provided us with targets to focus new therapies on. *Second-generation prognostic factors* include Ki67, cancer cell surface receptors for hormones, and Her2. The Ki67 is a test that demonstrates the percentage of cancer cells that are entering cell division (*mitosis*) and is therefore a test of *proliferation*. Results of this test should correspond to the mitotic score in the modified Bloom-Richardson.

Second-generation tests not only help oncologists identify women who need adjuvant therapy, they also help select the therapy that is most appropriate. For example, patients whose tumors show a high Ki67 score will have a good response to chemotherapy. We know this from research trials with preoperative (*neoadjuvant*) treatment. Tumors with hormone receptors on their cell surface respond to tamoxifen and the aromatase inhibitors. Cancers that overexpress the Her2 oncogene respond to targeted therapies, such as Herceptin and lapatinib, that are directed at the Her2 pathways.

We are now entering the most exciting and revolutionary era of breast cancer treatment with the introduction of *third-generation prognostic tests*, also called *genomic testing* and *molecular profiling*. These new tests can actually identify genes and proteins that are responsible for the development and spread of cancer. As discussed earlier, the two commercially available tests, Oncotype DX and MammaPrint, both use a technique known as *reverse transcription-polymerase chain reaction* (*RT-PCR*). This test is performed on cancer cells and identifies abnormal genes associated with the malignant processes of *proliferation, invasion*, and *angiogenesis*. Like the second-generation tests, these analyses also have the potential to help oncologists select therapies targeted at individual patient tumors. I predict that by the time I write the next edition of this book, third-generation prognostic tests will be the area where we see the most progress in breast cancer cure.

The critical questions for you and your treating doctors to discuss are: Do you need systemic therapy, based on the prognostic factors of your cancer? What are the risks of systemic treatment? Is the potential *benefit* of an increased cure rate worth the *risks* of treatment? This is

	Prognostic factors	Your results
First Generation	Tumor size	
	Lymph node involvement	
	Tumor grade	
Second Generation	Ki67 (proliferative rate)	
	Hormone receptors	
	Her2	
Third Generation	Oncotype DX	
	MammaPrint	

Table 6.1

Prognostic factors worksheet

not an easy discussion. Before making an informed decision, which takes into account your unique situation, you must understand what the treatment entails (including potential long-term side effects) and weigh that against the increase in cure rate.

Table 6.1 is a worksheet that lists the three generations of prognostic tests. Using this worksheet and, with the help of your oncologist, you can determine your risk of systemic spread. The flip side is to examine your cure rate with local control alone. There is a computer program available known as *Adjuvant Online* that can help you and your physician in making these decisions. You will probably access this very valuable program with your oncologist during your treatment planning visit. Coupled with the risk assessment will be an estimation of benefit from both chemotherapy and hormonal therapy. I think this tool is very valuable for risk/benefit assessment, but you must remember that it is just a tool.

Figure 6.1 shows how physicians decide on a *systemic treatment plan*

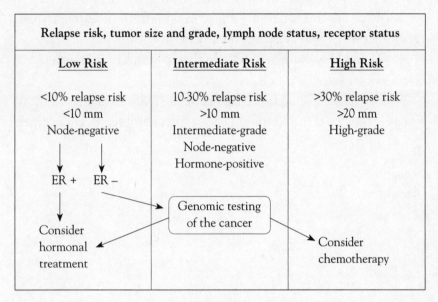

Figure 6.1

Making the decision for systemic treatment

for women with invasive breast cancer. It is critical that they select women who will benefit from these therapies and spare those women who will have a high cure rate with local control alone.

Your age is also an important factor in the decision process. In my experience older patients tend to decline chemotherapy when the survival benefit is small (10 percent or less). The survival benefit must be weighed against the potential side effects. We find that women will accept temporary reversible side effects for an increased chance of cure. Unfortunately, some of the currently used agents can cause permanent damage. These side effects are rare, but need to be carefully considered with your oncologist. The following are questions and considerations:

CHECKPOINTS

1. What is my cure rate with local control?
2. What is my increased cure rate with systemic control?

3. What are the potential long-term side effects of systemic treatment that will affect my quality of life?
4. Would I benefit from systemic therapy prior to surgery?

Now in the following two chapters we are ready to discuss adjuvant systemic therapy directed toward each of the four breast cancer types.

7

·······

❧

Chemotherapy

If you are reading this chapter because your oncologist is recommending chemotherapy as part of your treatment plan, keep in mind that there has been tremendous progress over the last thirty years in drug development, selection of treatment regimen, and management of side effects.

In the early 1980s the medical community determined that a course of chemotherapy improved the cure rate in women with invasive breast cancer. Based on early research trials, most women with invasive breast cancer of at least 1 centimeter or more were offered chemotherapy. In the last ten years we have begun to identify which women will most likely benefit from chemotherapy, and tailor chemotherapy treatment based on the individual woman's situation. There continues to be progress in these areas as we discover new genomic tests that assess the risk of systemic relapse. We are much better at matching women with the optimal therapy they need based on age, cancer stage, and tumor type, and good progress has been made in sorting out which drugs are better and at what dosage intensity.

I think of *adjuvant* chemotherapy as insurance *in case cells have escaped into the system*. With proper selection of drug regimens matched to individual patients, chemotherapy can greatly improve a woman's chance of surviving a breast cancer. How much do the odds improve? We are now approaching a 50 *percent increase in cure rate* in women whose risk of systemic spread (*metastasis*) is high enough to justify the use of chemotherapy. (This can be a complex process as discussed in chapter 6.)

The first decision to be made is whether you will receive chemotherapy, based on your own particular situation. If so, the next decision is the type of chemotherapy regimen you will be given, including the number of treatments and the time interval between them.

Chemotherapy works by killing cells that are dividing. Breast cancer cells are different from noncancer cells in that they divide on a regular interval. The shorter the interval, the more vulnerable or sensitive the cancer cells are to chemotherapy. In addition, cancer cells often lack the ability to repair the damage done to them by the chemotherapy agents, while normal cells retain their normal repair mechanisms.

A number of new agents are under investigation that interfere with DNA repair. One group of agents, known as *PARP inhibitors* (they inhibit the enzyme *Poly ADP ribose polymerase*), are being combined with *cytotoxic* (cell-killing) chemotherapy, and the results are very promising. Healthy cells can use the PARP enzyme to repair themselves and live out their normal life cycle. But *cancer cells* may also use the PARP enzyme to repair DNA damage, thus extending their uncontrolled growth. PARP inhibitor agents are being developed as a part of new clinical trials that will be available in the very near future. The first trials will be for women who are positive for the BRCA1 or BRCA2 gene and for women with triple-negative (basal type) breast cancer. This is because women who have inherited one of these mutations in their breast cells are already missing one of a pair of important DNA repair genes. The PARP inhibitors make the cancer cells extremely vulnerable to chemotherapy and unable to repair themselves from the damage. There is also evidence that some types of triple-negative breast cancer are sensitive to PARP inhibitors.

Chemotherapy agents work at different points in the dividing cell. In order to target multiple points within the cancer cell, the oncologist may combine different drugs to obtain added or even synergistic effects. The drug combinations have been developed through clinical trials and include drugs given at the same time or sequentially, one after the other, depending on their unique behavior (or mechanism) and shared toxicity.

As we are sorting out the internal pathways inside the cancer cell that differ from the normal cell, we are finding new "targets" to focus on, inviting development of new drugs directed specifically at these targets. Using techniques that can identify and measure increased or decreased proteins in the malignant cell, we can select drug regimens that greatly enhance our ability to kill the cancer. As I mentioned in the previous chapter, this is an extremely exciting and important area of breast cancer research.

In the past we identified women to receive chemotherapy based on the appearance of the cancer under the microscope and the stage of the cancer at diagnosis. Fourteen years ago, when we wrote the first edition of this manual, *all* women who had cancer that had spread to lymph nodes were given chemotherapy. There has been real progress over the past fourteen years; we now have improved tools to identify those women who will benefit from the variety of systemic treatments. In addition, we have new and better drugs designed to target cancer cells and be less toxic to the patient's normal cells. I believe development of the new classifications for breast cancer, based on genomic typing (discussed in chapter 3), is a major advance in helping us select appropriate treatment that is specific to a patient's individual cancer type. In the following section we discuss chemotherapy regimens for each of the new classifications. To this end, you will need to know your breast cancer type.

Systemic Therapy by Breast Cancer Type

1. Luminal A Breast Cancer

As discussed in chapter 3, Luminal A cancers are *well differentiated*; that is, they closely resemble normal tissue cells. Luminal A cancers are also

Luminal A breast cancer	
Cell type	Ductal
Grade	Low
Ki67 (proliferative rate)	Low
Spread to lymph nodes	Low
Hormone receptor status	Positive

Table 7.1

Luminal A Breast Cancer

low-proliferative cancers, meaning they are not likely to grow and increase in numbers rapidly. They are routinely found on screening mammograms and are positive for hormone receptors on their cell surface. On the newer commercially available tests such as Oncotype DX or MammaPrint, these cancers receive a *low-risk* score. Luminal A cancers tend to stay localized and seldom spread into the bloodstream. (See Table 7.1.)

Chemotherapy agents (drugs that kill cells based on cell division) have little effect or benefit on this cancer type. Because Luminal A cancer cells have hormone receptors on their surface, the treatment of choice will target these receptors, interfering with the cell's dependence on estrogen. Researchers in the past investigated possible therapies that would target the progesterone receptors on cancer cells; however, results to date have not led to effective targeted therapies. (We discuss targeted hormonal treatment in detail in chapter 8.)

2. Luminal B Breast Cancer

Luminal B cancers are positive for hormone receptors on their cell surface, but under the microscope they are a higher grade. Grade is measured using the *modified Bloom-Richardson* (MBR) scoring system (described in chapter 4). Under the old classification Luminal B cancers can be either *lobular* or *ductal*. The *Ki67 proliferative marker* is intermediate to high, and the *mitotic score* on the MBR is 2 or 3. Lumi-

Luminal B breast cancer	
Cell type	Ductal & lobular
Grade	Intermediate & high
Ki67 (proliferative rate)	Intermediate & high
Spread to lymph nodes	Intermediate
Hormone receptor status	Positive

Table 7.2
Luminal B breast cancer

nal B cancers are more aggressive than Luminal A and spread more readily to the lymph nodes and bloodstream. (See Table 7.2.)

Chemotherapy does provide some survival benefit (increased survival rate) in these cancers. But before you proceed with chemotherapy, you must carefully analyze its risks and benefits for your unique situation. High Ki67 proliferative scores and lymph node spread predict that chemotherapy will be beneficial. For Luminal B cancers that have not spread to the lymph nodes, the genomic tests Oncotype DX and MammaPrint are helpful to predict the value of chemotherapy. These two tests may even be helpful where there is limited spread to lymph nodes. Luminal B cancer that is less than 1 centimeter (10 mm) with *no* spread to lymph node(s) has a less than 10 percent risk of spreading into the bloodstream. In this case the survival benefit from chemotherapy is small, and hormonal treatment is the preferred therapy.

For women with Luminal B cancers where chemotherapy would be considered, the standard drug regimen is controversial. Clinical research trials and new understanding of how chemotherapy works demonstrate that drugs classified as *anthracyclines* (doxorubicin, Adriamycin, epirubicin) are minimally beneficial and produce a significant toxicity. Currently, the standard regimen consists of an *alkylating agent* (cyclophosphamide, Cytoxan) and a *taxane* (docetaxel, paclitaxel) with or without an anthracycline. We now believe there is enough evidence against the use of anthracyclines for this type of cancer; therefore we do not recommend their use.

Not only do Luminal B cancers have positive hormone receptors on their cell surface; there is also a tendency to lose the progesterone receptor. Following chemotherapy, hormonal therapy is used. For cancers that do not require chemotherapy, hormone therapy is prescribed (see chapter 8).

3. Basal Type (Triple-Negative) Breast Cancer

The third type of invasive breast cancer is termed *basal* or *triple-negative* because the cell surface lacks receptors for estrogen, progesterone, and Her2. It accounts for between 10 to 20 percent of newly diagnosed breast cancer. (See Table 7.3 for a summary of its characteristics.)

Due to the *high-proliferative* (fast-growing) nature of triple-negative breast cancers, they tend to be very sensitive to *cytotoxic chemotherapies* (chemicals that are toxic to cells). They may also lack DNA repair genes that would allow the cells to counter the lethal effects of chemotherapy. This is particularly true in women who are positive for the BRCA mutation.

Numerous chemotherapy drugs are used in triple-negative breast cancer (see Figure 7.1). Clinical trials suggest that shortening the amount of time between chemotherapy treatments may be beneficial in these cancers. This type of therapy has been termed *dose-dense* because the

Basal or triple-negative breast cancer	
Cell type	Ductal
Grade	Intermediate to high
Ki67 (proliferative rate)	High
Spread to lymph nodes	Frequent
Hormone receptor status	Negative

Table 7.3

Basal, or triple-negative breast cancer

Chemotheraphy drugs used for triple-negative breast cancer

cyclophosphamide

taxanes
- Taxol (paclitaxel)
- Taxotere (docetaxel)
- Abraxane (nab-paclitaxel)

doxorubicin (adriamycin)

cisplatin

PARP inhibitors*

antiangiogenesis (bevacizumab)*

*investigational

Figure 7.1

Chemotherapy drugs used for triple-negative breast cancer

standard drug regimen is delivered but in a shorter period of time. Breast cancer researchers are testing new treatment regimens by adding newly developed drugs that prevent DNA repair (*PARP inhibitors*) or *antiangiogenesis drugs* (substances that stop tumors from making new blood vessels) like bevacizumab (Avastin) to standard chemotherapy protocols.

Because triple-negative breast cancers grow rapidly and are found more often in younger women, the cancer is commonly discovered as a breast mass or lump. Once the tumor is imaged and biopsied, many women receive chemotherapy *prior* to surgery (*neoadjuvant*), as will be discussed later in this chapter. The sequence of treatment is important to discuss with your treatment team. The neoadjuvant approach also allows for new drugs to be tested on the cancer before it is removed from the breast. A positive response in the breast cancer and lymph nodes indicates that the chosen chemotherapy is effective and predicts that *micrometastatic* disease is also being eradicated. At this point you should consider asking your medical team if you are eligible for a clinical trial.

Triple-negative breast cancer has gotten a bad rap in the community perhaps because, unlike the case with Luminal A, B, and Her2 types, there are no targeted therapies currently available. The good news, as stated previously, is that triple-negative cancers are very sensitive to chemotherapy agents. We see this when a patient diagnosed with a triple-negative, palpable breast mass receives chemotherapy prior to surgery. After only one or two treatments there is often dramatic shrinkage of the mass, and in some cases the cancer disappears completely. Researchers are studying the molecular pathways within the triple-negative cancer cells to discover the different mechanisms that will allow development of better and more targeted therapies.

If a woman with triple-negative breast cancer goes three years beyond treatment without a recurrence, she is most likely cured. (We cannot say the same for those women who have Luminal A or Luminal B cancers.)

The gene analysis that identifies the basal type is currently on track to become commercially available. We have discovered that a handful of patients with basal type breast cancer are in fact not triple-negative but have some hormone or Her2 activity. Regardless of this positivity this basal type still behaves like triple-negative cancers and responds to treatments developed for triple-negative.

4. Her2-Positive Breast Cancer

The most progress in breast cancer research and treatment has been made with the type known as *Her2* (human epidermal growth factor receptor 2). These cancers have a protein receptor on their cell surface called the *Her2 receptor*, which has become a target for new cancer therapies. The prognosis for this type of breast cancer has greatly improved due to the development of agents that target the Her2 receptor and the Her2 molecular pathway within the cell.

This type of breast cancer accounts for about 15 percent of all newly diagnosed breast cancers. As discussed in chapter 3, Her2 cancers tend to be aggressive and spread to the bloodstream early, requiring systemic treatment to prevent a relapse.

It is critically important to identify Her2-positive breast cancers so

Her2-positive breast cancer	
Cell type	Ductal
Grade	High
Spread to lymph nodes	Frequent
Ki67 (proliferative rate)	High
Cell surface receptors	Her2-positive, ER/PR negative or positive

Table 7.4

Her2-positive breast cancer

appropriate treatment regimens can be used. Most women initially have a needle biopsy of the cancer. A special antibody stain directed at Her2 receptors on the cell surface is applied to the tissue biopsy sample. This staining, called *immunohistologic chemical staining* (IHC), is the first phase of testing. If no staining (0) or minimal staining (1) occurs on the cell surface, the cancer is Her2-negative. If the cancer cells show a strong staining (3), the cancer is positive for Her2. Intermediate-staining (2) cancers require further testing. There are several technologies available for this additional testing, but the *fluorescent in situ hybridization* (FISH) is the most widely used. This test measures the number of Her2 proteins that appear in the cell nucleus using a fluorescent antibody stain. Another method to determine if IHC 2+ tumors truly are Her2-positive relies on RT-PCR technology to measure intracellular Her2 RNA.

Patients with Her2-positive *invasive* breast cancer, as determined by IHC (3), FISH, or RT-PCR testing, have increased cure rates when given chemotherapy combined with an antibody to the Her2 receptor on the cancer cell surface called *trastuzumab* (*Herceptin*).

The discovery of Herceptin has been perhaps the most important event in breast cancer treatment history. In 2008 the Food and Drug Administration (FDA) approved the use of Herceptin for the treatment

Her2 treatment regimens

Adriamycin (*doxorubicin*) + Cytoxin (*cylophosphamide*) × 4 treatments
   ➡ Taxotere (docetaxol) + Herceptin × 4 treatments
   ➡ Herceptin for 12 months **TOTAL**

Taxotere (*docetaxol*) + carboplatin + Herceptin × 6 treatments   ➡ Herceptin for 12 months **TOTAL**

Figure 7.2

Her2 treatment regimens

of early breast cancer, based on several pivotal trials that compared cure rates for two groups of women with early-stage cancer: those treated with chemotherapy alone and those who received chemotherapy plus Herceptin. The increase in cure rate for the latter group was phenomenal. Treatment regimens based on these groundbreaking trials are outlined in Figure 7.2. After several months of Herceptin/chemotherapy combination, Herceptin alone is continued for a total of one year of treatment.

Herceptin works by binding to the Her2 receptors on the cell surface and interrupting the Her2 pathway within the cell, leading to cell death. While the exact mechanism is unclear, Herceptin appears to make the cell more sensitive to the effects of chemotherapy.

A number of new molecules have been discovered that disrupt the Her2 pathway inside the cell. Lapatinib (Tykerb) is the first of these treatment molecules to receive FDA approval for metastatic disease and is being tested in early breast cancer combined with Herceptin and chemotherapy. Other Her2-targeted therapies are currently in Phase 1 and Phase 2 trials and include TDM1 (discussed in the next paragraph), pertuzumab, and neratinib. It is very likely that these drugs will be in clinical trials for newly diagnosed Her2-positive breast cancer in the near future. Ask your oncologist if you are a candidate for one of these clinical trials.

With the use of Herceptin and Tykerb we have entered a "new era" of targeted treatments for breast cancer based on disruption of the *genomic message* within the cancer cell. These drugs are less toxic to normal cells than older traditional chemotherapies. Research will ultimately deliver many more of these new agents. Current research trials are combining Herceptin (trastuzumab) with a linked cytotoxic drug called DM1—the combination is called TDM1—and the results are very promising in the early phases. This molecule is delivered directly to the cancer cell and appears to have minimal toxicity to the noncancerous cells.

As in triple-negative breast cancer, Her2-positive cancers are fast growing and are often discovered as a palpable mass rather than from a mammogram. Women with this type of presentation are candidates for Herceptin-based chemotherapy prior to surgery, as will be discussed in the next section.

Preoperative (Neoadjuvant) Systemic Therapy

✂ The use of *preoperative systemic therapy* (*neoadjuvant*) has become standard for many women with newly discovered breast cancer. The traditional sequence of treatment has been surgery followed by *adjuvant systemic therapy* when needed. More recently, many women, based on information found through examination of the needle biopsy tissue, benefit from reversing this sequence so they receive systemic therapy *prior* to surgery.

There are four major advantages to administering chemotherapy prior to surgery. 1. Treatment can be initiated almost immediately to the whole body (breast cancer, lymph nodes, and/or bloodstream). 2. Most often this will result in less aggressive surgery to the breast and lymph node area. 3. The response to therapy can be directly observed with shrinkage of the primary cancer and any involved lymph nodes, which indicates that the correct drug regimen has been selected. 4. Patients that do not have a significant response will be identified and further study of their cancer may lead to different treatment with better survival.

Preoperative chemotherapy involves a period of twelve to twenty weeks, and patients who are good candidates for this treatment regimen will almost always respond with shrinkage of the cancer. During this phase of treatment, the patient and medical team can explore surgical options and consider genetic testing if indicated. In the past, some women may have rushed into surgery unnecessarily and possibly to their disadvantage. If your cancer has one or more of the following character-istics, you are a good candidate for preoperative chemotherapy.

1. Invasive cancer that is palpable or larger than 2 centimeters
2. Positive lymph nodes on physical exam or by imaging
3. Intermediate- or high-grade histology (high modified Bloom-Richardson score: 2 or 3)
4. Elevated Ki67
5. Luminal B cancers that have the above characteristics
6. Triple-negative or Her2-positive cancers

You should discuss whether you are a good candidate for preop-erative chemotherapy with your treatment team. Patients with large, low-grade hormone-positive tumors occasionally receive *preoperative hormonal therapy*. This approach is more common in Europe, but its use in North America is increasing. The response is slower, over three to six months, and for some women this allows for better timing of surgery. Studies indicate that there is no loss in survival rates with this approach.

The use of preoperative systemic therapy in the research setting has been very important to our progress. We know from a number of studies that women who achieve a complete response following preoperative therapy (no cancer remains at the time of surgery) have a very high cure rate. If by adding a new, promising, and safe treatment to the cur-rent *best regimen*, a higher complete response is achieved, we have made progress. The old way of comparing results from different regimens administered after surgery required years to determine a difference in relapse and survival rates. Again, ask your doctors if you qualify for this type of research trial.

The Risks of Chemotherapy

✄ The majority of women with newly diagnosed breast cancer will be cured. To achieve this outcome, women at highest risk of systemic spread will be advised to undergo some form of chemotherapy as previously discussed—but at what cost?

As noted earlier, most, if not all, women are willing to undergo temporary, reversible side effects for a good chance of increased cure. Temporary side effects (*risks*) from chemotherapy can include hair loss, fatigue, nausea, diarrhea, mental fogginess, and increased chance of infection. However, with the new protective treatment regimens that have been developed, many women will suffer none of these side effects. The one problem that still remains is temporary hair loss. (See chapter 10.)

A major issue with chemotherapy is the risk of permanent damage that might affect future health. While I believe the risk of permanent lifelong side effects is small, it needs to be addressed. Fertility and premature menopause are the biggest concerns for young women. Most women in their thirties and early forties will maintain hormone function and fertility; however, there is some increased risk of ovarian failure with chemotherapy, and this issue should be explored with your oncologist before beginning treatment. Hormones can be replaced, and egg harvesting is an additional option. In my experience most young women undergoing chemotherapy will regain ovarian function after treatment is completed. This appears to be age dependent; the closer a woman is to menopause, the higher the risk of premature ovarian failure. If you are a young woman with newly diagnosed breast cancer, you might consider scheduling a consultation with a fertility expert.

Although the risk of secondary cancer from chemotherapy does exist, it is very remote. The anthracyclines (doxorubicin and epirubicin) have a small increased risk of acute leukemia, but they are being utilized less in breast cancer treatment. *Neuropathy*—damage to the peripheral nerves (nerves outside the brain or spinal cord)—occurs with the taxanes and is usually reversible. Neuropathy is usually manifested by numbness in the fingers and toes and a change in taste that many women describe as muted, bland, or metallic.

The issue of mental or cognitive dysfunction resulting from chemotherapy is a topic much discussed in support groups and on the Internet. This issue is complex because it involves a number of factors: effects of chemotherapy on the ovaries, resulting in decreased hormone levels; stress; drugs used for sedation, anxiety, or sleep, and/or to prevent side effects. The term *chemonesia* has emerged to describe this mental dysfunction. I believe this side effect is temporary and is completely reversible. Most women taking adjuvant or neoadjuvant chemotherapy are able to continue their lives fairly normally.

The way patients react to chemotherapy varies considerably. Fatigue seems to be the major issue. Women want to know if they can continue to work while on chemotherapy, and the answer depends on the treatment regimen used and the individual's job requirements and stress. Because chemotherapy drugs negatively affect immune function, reducing the body's ability to fight infection, women often ask if they can go out in public or be around small children. Our advice is to avoid individuals who are obviously sick, but you don't need to make major modifications in how you live your life. The truth is, most infections that occur during chemotherapy come from bacteria that inhabit your skin or gastrointestinal tract. Fever is often the first sign of infection, and your oncologist will give you instructions to follow if a fever develops during chemotherapy.

Chemotherapy affects the *bone marrow* (blood-producing cells), causing *low white blood cell* counts (which compromises the body's ability to fight infection) and *anemia* (low red blood cell counts, which sap energy). Both can be corrected by using special drugs that stimulate the bone marrow to recover more quickly. Many chemotherapy regimens will include the addition of these medicines to prevent infection and fatigue. (These issues will be further discussed in chapter 10.)

CHECKPOINTS

1. Will I have a survival advantage with the addition of chemotherapy, and if so, how much?
2. Am I a candidate to receive chemotherapy before surgery?
3. What is the risk involved in the chemotherapy that is recommended for me? Has my oncologist explained short-term reversible side effects as compared to potential long-term, permanent effects?
4. Am I eligible for a clinical trial?

8

······

❧

Hormonal Therapy

We have known for many years that most breast cancer is somehow regulated by hormones and that certain hereditary factors and/or life experiences can increase breast cancer risk. For example, the longer a woman menstruates, the higher her risk of developing breast cancer. Pregnancy with long periods of breast-feeding *decreases* the total number of menstrual periods, and therefore may protect against breast cancer. The first randomized clinical trial in postmenopausal women using the combination of progesterone and estrogen (Prempro) indicated that there is a slight *increased* risk of breast cancer in women who use hormone replacement therapy (HRT). In the same study, women using estrogen alone (those who were posthysterectomy) showed no increase in breast cancer risk. This suggests that perhaps the combination of estrogen with progesterone is problematic. Years before the introduction of chemotherapy and hormone therapy as breast cancer treatments, we learned that removing a women's ovaries or adrenal glands could result in the regression or complete disappearance of metastatic disease. This discovery identified the relationship between estrogen and breast cancer and led to the development of drugs that treat breast cancer (tamoxifen and aromatase inhibitors)

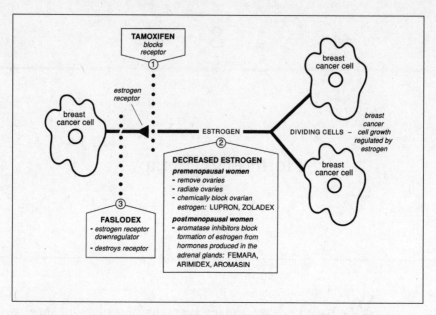

Figure 8.1

Regulating estrogen exposure to affect breast cancer cell growth

and reduce breast cancer risk (tamoxifen, Evista [raloxifene], and Aromasin [exemestane]).

The growth of a breast cancer cell is affected by exposure to estrogen (see Figure 8.1). It is possible to regulate this process through three different mechanisms.

1. Block the estrogen receptors so that estrogen cannot attach itself to the receptor sites on the cell surface and stimulate growth (tamoxifen-like drugs or SERMs).
2. Decrease estrogen levels in premenopausal women by suppressing ovarian production through the use of the drug Lupron or Zoladex. In postmenopausal women aromatase inhibitors (AIs) are used to suppress adrenal estrogen production.
3. Eliminate the estrogen receptors on the cell surface (the drug Faslodex or SERDs).

Selective Estrogen Receptor Modulators (SERMs)

✒ Human female cells that contain receptors for estrogen or estrogen-like molecules are found in the breast, uterus, vagina, ovaries, brain, and skin. A class of medications known as Selective Estrogen Receptor Modulators (SERMS) have been specifically designed to attach to these cell surface receptors and act like keys to turn cellular function on or off. Tamoxifen is a SERM.

Estrogen attaches to receptors on breast cells and stimulates them to grow and divide. This action is controlled by a network of protein messengers contained within the cell. The drug tamoxifen was developed to attach to the estrogen receptor site and turn this mechanism off. In the case of breast cancer cells that contain estrogen receptors, tamoxifen may actually send the cell into a programmed death cycle. Tamoxifen is taken orally like other hormones. In spite of *turning off* normal breast cells and breast cancer cells, it can also act like estrogen on other cells, with positive effects such as preventing bone loss and lowering cholesterol (see Table 8.1).

There have been long-term studies demonstrating that tamoxifen increases the cure rate for women with localized breast cancer, but controversy still continues to surround its use. Part of the controversy stems from a national clinical trial conducted to determine whether tamoxifen can prevent primary breast cancer in high-risk *unaffected* women. As a result of this trial, tamoxifen received heavy scrutiny due to reported side effects, including increased risk of uterine cancer and blood clots. I believe that this risk is small and acceptable when compared with the benefit received. In most cases, women who are given tamoxifen to increase their cure rate accept potential or real side effects more readily than women given the drug for breast cancer prevention. This prevention study and a subsequent study comparing tamoxifen to raloxifene (a SERM closely related to tamoxifen) showed a reduction in breast cancer occurrence in high-risk women. In fact, raloxifene showed an equivalent reduction in breast cancer occurrence with fewer side effects, particularly a lower risk of uterine cancer. It should be noted that both tamoxifen and raloxifene reduce the incidence of breast cancer in high-risk women if taken for five years, but to date there is no reduction in breast cancer deaths due to treatment regimens using these SERMS. Raloxifene has proven effective for *preventing* breast cancer in *postmenopausal* women but has not been studied for treating existing breast cancer. Tamoxifen remains the gold-standard SERM for those patients already diagnosed.

There is absolutely no question that tamoxifen is an extremely valuable treatment for women with breast cancer, and most women tolerate its modest side effects without major problems. Trials suggest that five years of tamoxifen therapy significantly reduces the systemic recurrence of breast cancer, but an additional five years adds only expense and potential increased risk of uterine cancer with no change in cure rate. The current thinking, with rare exceptions, is to stop tamoxifen after five years of treatment for primary breast cancer. Not all breast cancers respond to tamoxifen, however; prediction of response can be determined and is based on the presence of estrogen and progesterone receptors in the primary tumor (chapter 4).

When tamoxifen trials were launched over twenty years ago, we did not fully understand how tamoxifen worked, but today, with our increased knowledge of molecular pathways within the cell, its mechanism of action is much better understood. In the beginning, we thought that tamoxifen blocked estrogen production by the ovaries, which we now know is not the case. The ovaries produce the majority of estrogen normally, while the adrenal glands produce much lesser amounts. Estrogen affects multiple organs, including the breast, uterus, skin, brain, liver, and vagina. Tamoxifen was believed to have *anti-estrogen* effects as long as women were taking it. The effects were on both cancer cells and estrogen-sensitive cells in various tissues. If women were to stop taking tamoxifen, we thought the blockade would be removed and all the preventive good it had done would be reversed. If this were the case, tamoxifen would be called a *static agent*. An analogy is a static antibiotic, which paralyzes bacteria, allowing white blood cells to come along and gobble them up. The counterpart is the cidal antibiotic, which kills bacteria on its own and does not need white blood cells to complete the job. We thought that tamoxifen was a static cancer drug because it put cancer cells to rest but couldn't finish them off.

Now, after a number of years of follow-up, we consider tamoxifen to be a cidal agent. Tamoxifen actually binds to the hormone receptor on the surface of the cancer cell, preventing estrogen from attaching and stimulating the cell to divide. We have learned that tamoxifen is not static at all but appears to directly disrupt the cancer cell's life cycle. Since breast cancers are heterogeneous, they are not all constructed in the same way: about 60 percent of breast cancers contain hormone receptors; the others do not. Tamoxifen appears to be helpful to women who have estrogen and progesterone hormone receptors on their cell surfaces. However, within a given breast cancer, there may be cells that have more hormone receptors than others. Thus tamoxifen may be only partly effective. It is also possible that, over time, a population of cells that are hormone receptor–positive may even evolve and become hormone receptor–negative and thus resistant to hormonal therapy. In theory, this may be why some women who receive a combination of chemotherapy and tamoxifen have a better response than if they received either treatment alone. Usually, when chemotherapy and tamoxifen are used, they are given sequentially (one after the other); chemotherapy, which kills off cells that are potentially resistant to tamoxifen, is given first, followed by tamoxifen, which can then target the hormone-sensitive cancer cells that may be less susceptible to chemotherapy.

Side effects of tamoxifen are very different from those of cytotoxic chemotherapy. Tamoxifen's side effects are primarily hormonal. For women close to menopause, tamoxifen produces more menopausal-like symptoms. (Table 8.1 shows some of the expected effects of estrogen versus tamoxifen on estrogen-receptive tissues.) Women who seem to have the most difficulty with tamoxifen are *perimenopausal* (about

to begin menopause) and menopausal women on hormone replacement therapy (HRT) who go off their HRT because of their recent
breast cancer diagnoses. Older women who are not on replacement
hormones have few problems starting and taking tamoxifen. Likewise,
younger *premenopausal* women often have few side effects and usually
tolerate the treatment well. Tamoxifen may interfere with ovulation,
and young women may occasionally experience irregular periods and
increased incidence of ovarian cysts.

The major potential toxic effect of tamoxifen is to the uterus. A
small percentage of women have endometrial thickening, a stimulation to the glandular lining of the uterus, which, if left unchecked,
can become cancerous. The chance of uterine malignancy as a result
of taking tamoxifen is small, less than 1 percent, but routine pelvic
examination should be performed. Uterine cancer is extremely rare in
women under the age of fifty-five and presents very early with postmenopausal vaginal bleeding. Uterine cancer is almost always curable

	Tamoxifen	Estrogen	Explanation
Breast	–	+++	Estrogen stimulates breast epithelial proliferation.
Uterus	++	++++	Estrogen stimulates uterine lining slightly more than tamoxifen.
Skin	+	++	Estrogen increases tissue moisture.
Vagina	–	++	Estrogen stimulates vaginal proliferation and lubrication.
Bone	++	++	Both tamoxifen and estrogen help retain bone calcium.
Hot Flashes	–	++	Estrogen reduces hot flashes.

Table 8.1

Effects of estrogen and tamoxifen on female cells

with hysterectomy, and the threat of uterine cancer should not, as a general rule, dissuade women from taking tamoxifen if the survival benefit justifies its use.

A major potential side effect of tamoxifen is the development of blood clots. Fortunately, this serious type of venous blood clot (pulmonary embolus) is rare and should not be the reason to avoid tamoxifen use. Women with a family history of venous thrombosis should be tested for Factor V (Leiden) deficiency. This common hereditary hypercoagulability disorder increases an individual's risk of venous blood clots. The risk increases even more for women taking tamoxifen. Patients with serious clotting disorders may be better off choosing an alternative hormone therapy such as one of the aromatase inhibitors.

Potentially uncomfortable side effects with tamoxifen can include vaginal dryness, hot flashes, and mild weight gain. These symptoms can be managed using remedies that include medications, natural products, and/or herbs. Women often ask, "Are these side effects worth the benefit gained by taking tamoxifen?" The answer is—*absolutely!* The potential survival benefit for those on tamoxifen is on average 10 to 25 percent greater than it is for those women who do not take it; as noted earlier, the uterine cancer risk is less than 1 percent, and this type of cancer can be easily monitored and treated.

Recent results from clinical trials indicate that a small percentage of women are unable to metabolize tamoxifen appropriately because they lack an enzyme CYP2D6 in their liver and receive no benefit from this hormone regimine. These women can be identified by a simple blood test to determine adequate CYP2D6 activity. Only about 5 percent of the female population tests positive for this deficiency, with the abnormality moderately higher in Asian women. Toremifene, a SERM very similar to tamoxifen, is not affected by CYP2D6 and is therefore the alternative of choice in these cases.

Tamoxifen was the first SERM developed, and we have almost thirty years of experience using the drug. As mentioned, another SERM, raloxifene, has been shown to prevent breast cancer in high-risk patients.

The goal is to develop the *perfect* SERM, one that prevents breast cancer (or treats it) without stimulating the uterus, is beneficial to the bones, and is good for lipid metabolism without causing hot flashes and other menopausal symptoms. The perfect SERM would be an excellent therapy for menopausal women seeking hormone replacement.

Tamoxifen is the best-studied cancer drug, not only for breast cancer but for all other cancers. More than thirty thousand women have participated in studies to prove the benefits of tamoxifen, which include: prevention of breast cancer, treatment of DCIS, treatment of early invasive breast cancer and more advanced breast cancer. For the majority of patients, when tamoxifen is recommended, the benefits far outweigh any risks.

The Aromatase Inhibitors (AIs)

✂ The second way to treat estrogen-positive breast cancer is to stop estrogen production from nonovarian sources such as the adrenal gland by using aromatase inhibitors.

After menopause, the adrenal gland becomes the major source for the production of estrogen. Hormones produced in the adrenal gland are converted into estrogen in the body's fat and muscle tissue by the aromatase enzyme. Research shows that aromatase inhibitors can block the aromatase enzyme so that estrogen is not produced. The use of aromatase-inhibiting drugs is so effective that there is greater than a 99 percent reduction in estrogen production in postmenopausal women.

Currently, there are three aromatase inhibitors (AIs) available: Arimidex (anastrazole), Femara (letrozole), and Aromasin (exemestane). These drugs were originally introduced to treat patients with advanced metastatic breast cancer and were shown to be equal to and in some studies more effective than tamoxifen, with fewer serious side effects. Over time they began to be used for earlier stages of breast disease. An important clinical trial, the ATAC Trial (Arimidex, Tamoxifen, Alone or in Combination), compared five years of tamoxifen use to five years of Arimidex use. Now, after almost ten years of follow-up, the results suggest that Arimidex is slightly more effective than tamoxifen in preventing breast cancer recurrence, although the difference is small, which demonstrates that both are effective. In addition, Arimidex does not cause uterine cancer or blood clots, which are the major serious potential side effects of tamoxifen. Arimidex can increase joint pain and seems to increase the risk of osteoporosis. If you are postmenopausal, this information provides you and your oncologist several treatment options to consider.

Recent studies show that women who switch to an AI after two to three years of tamoxifen use have a lower relapse rate than women who continue on tamoxifen for the full five years. Also, women who take Femara after five years of tamoxifen use have a lower rate of relapse than women who stop tamoxifen after five years and take nothing. The length of time that a postmenopausal woman should take an aromatase inhibitor is still unclear but could be for as much as ten to fifteen years. Of course, weighing the risks and benefits of treatment for that length of time will have to be determined by the patient and her physician. Other factors such as bone density and arthritic symptoms will factor into this decision.

Selective Estrogen Receptor Downregulators (SERDs)

✂ The third way to block estrogen-stimulated growth of the cancer cell is by decreasing or destroying the estrogen receptors on the cell surface. A new class of drugs called SERDs (Selective Estrogen Receptor Downregulators) appears to eliminate the function of the estrogen receptor. The first drug of this type, recently approved by the FDA for patients with metastatic breast cancer, is called Faslodex (fulvestrant) and may soon become a third adjuvant alternative. Faslodex is a once-a-month injection given into the muscle. It has very few side effects and certainly has the advantage over tamoxifen of not causing blood clots or uterine cancer, and for metastatic patients it appears to be equally effective as the aromatase inhibitors. It allows doctors to monitor patients by seeing them once a month for injection. Women do not have to take a daily pill. The disadvantage is having to come to the doctor's office once a month and getting a shot in the buttocks; plus it is expensive. It is now clear that there are options other than tamoxifen and that new and better treatments will be developed to take advantage of the estrogen sensitivity of breast cancer cells. It is my guess that very soon hormonal therapy and chemotherapy will be *tailored* for each patient based on her individual cancer-molecular profile, further improving cure rates while keeping side effects to a minimum.

Hormonal Therapy in the Premenopausal Patient

✂ The treatment of choice for premenopausal, hormone receptor–positive breast cancer patients is tamoxifen. For years we have known that there is a relationship between estrogen and breast cancer. Several recent studies, primarily from England and Europe, have shown that ovarian suppression (surgical or chemical) in some premenopausal women can be as effective as chemotherapy without the associated side effects of chemotherapy. The drugs Lupron and Zoladex turn off the production of ovarian estrogen in premenopausal women and provide a nonpermanent and nonsurgical option. A major question in breast cancer treatment research is whether the suppression of estrogen production provides an added benefit to chemotherapy, particularly in women under the age of forty. Study results have been inconclusive, causing this approach to fall outside the current standard treatment. The potential benefit must be weighed against the side effects of premature menopause, which include infertility, accelerated bone loss, and menopausal symptoms. Ovarian suppression during chemotherapy may help to preserve ovarian function once chemotherapy is completed, although this too is currently under investigation.

Ovarian suppression during chemotherapy for young women with estrogen-negative cancers may be helpful for those interested in preserving ovarian function and fertility. New technologies offering egg and embryo storage may be solutions to the issues of fertility in patients and couples. If you are a premenopausal woman, you need to discuss the issues of fertility and menopause with your oncologist, along with all the risks and benefits in the use of systemic treatment. There is no convincing data that pregnancy after breast cancer is detrimental to a patient's survival. Of course, this too is an important topic for you to discuss with your oncologist, particularly if your risk of recurrence is significant.

CHECKPOINTS

1. Does my pathology report indicate that my cancer is hormone receptor–positive?
2. Is tamoxifen a potential therapy in my case? If yes, will I be tested for CYP2D6?
3. What are the risks and benefits of taking tamoxifen?
4. Do I have a personal history of blood clots or a family history of clots that would make an alternative to tamoxifen (an aromatase inhibitor) a better choice?
5. Should I consider raloxifene or tamoxifen for breast cancer prevention?
6. If I am postmenopausal, should I take an aromatase inhibitor rather than tamoxifen?
7. If I am postmenopausal, should I embark on a course of aromatase therapy after five years of tamoxifen?
8. Would I benefit by suppressing my ovaries with Lupron or Zolodex?
9. If I am premenopausal, am I a candidate for chemical or surgical ovarian suppression with or without chemotherapy?

9
·······

❧

Radiation Therapy

R adiation is a local treatment added to surgical removal of
the breast cancer and is used to prevent local recurrence. It is administered by physician specialists known as radiation oncologists. Radiation therapy is usually given with a large machine called a *linear
accelerator* that generates a high-energy x-ray beam used to treat a
specific, well-defined area of the body, or it can be administered using
radioactive seeds temporarily placed in the cancer site. Radiation affects
the tissue cells beneath the directed beam of x-rays. Cells that are
dividing are more affected by radiation than resting cells. Although
both cancer and normal cells are damaged by radiation, cancer cells,
because they are actively dividing, are most affected. In addition, normal cells have a greater ability than cancer cells to repair themselves
following radiation exposure. Radiation puts cancer cells into a cell
death cycle called *apoptosis*, a cycle that occurs the next time the cancer cell divides.

Many of our patients do not clearly understand the role that radiation therapy plays in the overall treatment plan. For instance, some
wonder why radiation is necessary if a breast cancer has been removed
by a *wide local excision* (WLE) with *clear margins*. In spite of local
removal, about 30 percent of women will relapse without radiation

therapy, whereas 5 percent or less who receive radiation will relapse. Pathologists can have trouble determining if there is a clear margin of normal tissue surrounding the cancer because it is often difficult to identify minuscule amounts of cancer cells. There may also be "skip" areas between the main tumor and very small, hard-to-detect satellite cancer nodules in the immediate vicinity. Therefore, in spite of clear margins, extremely small tumor cells may be resting on the outside of the surgical margins. In addition, cells may have traveled through the breast duct system and come to rest outside of the surgical site. Radiation is important because it has a good chance of destroying those random cancer cells.

Radiation to the chest surface is sometimes also recommended following mastectomy if the cancer is large, has extended to or through the surgical margins, or if multiple lymph nodes are involved with cancer. The addition of radiation in these situations reduces the incidence of local recurrence considerably.

Is radiation always necessary? If we could pick the 70 to 80 percent of women who would not have a local recurrence, we could avoid radiation in the majority of cases. Unfortunately, this is not so easy to do. If the cancer is small, with a large clear margin of uninvolved tissue, and if there is no local involvement in the lymph nodes or extensive DCIS, one might consider observation alone and no radiation.

Studies also indicate that a woman's age may be an important contributing factor for risk of local recurrence if radiation therapy is not administered. Dr. Umberto Veronesi, a world-renowned Italian breast surgeon, reported results from a study in which women with small T1 breast cancers (less than 20 mm) received wide local excision with clear surgical margins. Each woman was then randomly assigned to either *postoperative radiation* or *no radiation*. Women over the age of sixty had less than a 5 percent recurrence rate without radiation! Younger women had a higher local recurrence rate without radiation for reasons that are not clear. These findings have led to further studies in the United States confirming that older women (over the age of seventy) with early breast cancer can be spared radiation particularly if they are receiving hormonal therapy.

The typical course of radiation is daily treatment for twenty-five to thirty sessions. There is good reason to give such extended, prolonged treatment. A long string of short, individual treatments causes less damage to normal tissues, allowing them to repair completely, while increasing the progressive lethal damage to cancer cells. Recent studies suggest that it is safe and feasible to reduce the number of treatments to three weeks (fifteen total treatments). This course of radiation, called *hypofractionated* or *accelerated whole breast radiation*, reduces the number of treatments but increases the dose of each treatment. A large study in Canada of 2,500 women who received the reduced number of treatments showed no difference in local recurrence or survival rate with minor differences in skin reaction and fatigue.

Receiving radiation treatments involves several steps. First, you will have a consultation with the radiation oncologist, who will explain the risks and benefits of the treatment in detail. If radiation is to be part of treatment, the next step is a treatment planning session, called a simulation appointment, which can take one to two hours. Most radiation facilities use three-dimensional images from a special CT scanner called a *CT simulator* to plan treatments. During simulation, the radiation staff will position your body on the CT scanner in the appropriate treatment position—typically lying on your back with one or both arms resting over your head. They will use special devices such as an incline board or customized body pillow to maximize the comfort and reproducibility of your body position. To ensure accurate positioning prior to each radiation treatment, photographs are taken and small tattoos (the size of a beauty mark) and felt pen marks are placed on your skin. Stickers and tape may also be used to outline scars and protect ink marks. A CT scan of your body in the treatment position is then sent to the radiation planning computers. Over the next week, the radiation oncologist will work with a physics staff member to create a radiation treatment plan for you. The images from your simulation are used to target the radiation beam and calculate parameters for the linear accelerator to deliver the correct dose of radiation to your breast. When the treatment plan has been reviewed, approved, and has passed quality assurance checks, your radiation treatments will begin.

The daily treatment appointment is typically fifteen to thirty minutes. Most of that time is spent setting up and verifying the treatment position. The radiation beam is typically on for only one to two minutes from two to three different directions. As with a chest x-ray, there is no pain or heat when the radiation beam is passing through the breast. And you will not become radioactive or expose people to radiation from the treatments. The radiation treatments are given by highly trained technicians. Most women will see their radiation oncologist once a week for monitoring, but they should remember that their physician is always available for any special problems that may arise from the daily treatment. Don't hesitate to ask to see the doctor with any questions or concerns you may have.

If the margins around the cancer are surgically clear and the purpose of the radiation is to eradicate any microscopic cells that may have been left behind, twenty-five to thirty treatments to the entire breast or chest surface are usually adequate to achieve this goal. However, in younger women, or if the team has some question about margin involvement, an extra amount of radiation, called a *boost*, is given to the tumor area.

There are several methods of giving boosts. The most common involves the linear accelerator and consists of five to ten additional radiation treatments to the local surgical area using an electron beam. Unlike x-rays used to treat the entire breast, electrons penetrate less deeply into the breast tissue and can be used to target the superficial surgical scar and surgical site just beneath it. Sometimes x-rays are necessary for the boost if your surgical site is deep within a larger size breast.

An alternative method of boosting is the implantation of small seeds of radioactive material, called *iridium*, into the surgical area. These seeds remain in the breast for forty-eight to seventy-two hours. The surgeon implants these during a short surgical procedure; however, with the advent of the electron beam method of boosting, doctors are choosing to use these implants less frequently because of the hospitalization required, the expense, and patient discomfort.

There are side effects from radiation to the breast. It is usual to have some skin and breast tissue changes, such as redness and some inflammation that usually diminish over time. Ninety percent of women have an excellent cosmetic result after healing occurs. Ten percent have some added fibrous tissue, shrinkage of the breast, reduced skin elasticity, and breast sensitivity. There are treatments available that can be used to help facilitate healing and reduce the long-term effects of radiation.

Skin side effects must be taken into account when considering reconstruction after mastectomy. Radiation can cause problems with hardening of tissue around breast reconstruction implants or increased firmness in tissue transferred to the chest surface from a TRAM flap (discussed in chapter 11). You need to discuss with both the oncologist and the plastic surgeon the possibility of the need for radiation therapy. A consultation with a radiation oncologist prior to mastectomy may be helpful for understanding the potential radiation effects on a reconstructed breast. In some cases it is better to delay the breast reconstruction until after chemotherapy and radiation therapy so that all choices, with their associated risks and benefits, can best be reviewed with you. The majority of women who have reconstruction following radiation therapy will require the TRAM flap because of decreased skin elasticity and pliancy caused by the radiation. Some women will have reconstruction at the time of mastectomy, using temporary saline implants that are replaced with permanent implants in a second surgery. If radiation is needed after mastectomy, the second surgery will take place about six months after radiation is completed in order to minimize healing problems due to radiation.

As for other side effects, radiation does pose several. However, with modern techniques, the radiation beam is targeted more accurately and thereby avoids excessive radiation to the lungs and heart. The ribs beneath your treated breast may be tender for a year or longer. You may experience temporary fatigue and a mild depression of the white and red blood cell counts. You will not experience nausea or hair loss from your head.

When a woman needs both chemotherapy and radiation, chemotherapy is usually given first. This is because several of the chemotherapy agents raise the toxicity of the radiation and can cause increased skin changes if given along with radiation. Also, if the treatments were to be given at the same time, the bone marrow would suffer a greater impact, resulting in lower white blood cell counts, which can leave a patient more vulnerable to infection.

Many women express concern regarding radiation treatment and its ability to cause other cancers later in life. In order to understand the risk of this possibility, you should know the different sources and types of radiation that human beings are exposed to. Some are environmental, such as solar radiation, and are considered "natural," while others are man-made, such as those resulting from x-rays and imaging. It is true that in large doses, radiation is carcinogenic and can cause genetic mutation. This is often the result of partial injury to a cell that recovers and goes on to divide and pass on defects to offspring chromosomes.

These defects do not result from therapeutic radiation thanks to the p53 gene and other DNA repair genes. The p53 gene is in all cells in the body and appears to protect the cell from most of these mutations. Fortunately, if a cell is injured, the p53 gene prevents further cell division until repairs are made. It is amazing that the body has such self-healing potential.

A number of studies have been conducted to determine if there is an increased risk of a second cancer in patients treated with therapeutic radiation. Retrospective studies have looked at women receiving primary radiation for the treatment of breast cancer and the incidence of a second breast cancer and other types of malignancy. The bottom line is that there is a very *slight* increased risk of a second cancer as the result of radiation treatment. Women who have had radiation therapy have approximately a 1 percent chance of getting a second breast cancer from the treatment itself, compared with women who have not received radiation in the treatment of their breast cancer. Age seems to be a factor, and the highest risk occurs in women exposed to radiation at a young age. The risk for women over age forty appears to be negligible, but not zero.

The use of more limited radiation has been evaluated in clinical trials and is becoming more available and widely used. Because breast cancer tends to exist in a specific segment or quadrant and local recurrences are usually a centimeter or two from the site of the original cancer, it may be appropriate to limit the extent of radiation; by using radiation seeds or a radiation-filled balloon, the period of radiation exposure may be limited to only five days. This type of radiation, called *accelerated partial breast radiation*, appears to be appropriate for tumors that are unifocal (isolated to a single area in the breast), small (less than 3 cm), and far enough away from the skin to minimize skin injury. Patients with extensive in situ or lymphatic involvement are not good candidates for this accelerated partial breast radiation because of a higher risk of residual cancer away from the primary cancer. It is appropriate for you to discuss this treatment with your surgeon and radiation oncologist.

For women who choose to have WLE without radiation, there is an increased risk of local recurrence as stated above. A majority of these recurrences occur within one to two centimeters of the original tumor resection. This is why localized radiation reduces the incidence of local recurrence. Based on this knowledge, a number of clinical trials around the world have been conducted using a single treatment of radiation administered during the primary surgery. This technique, known as *intraoperative radiation* (IORT), was pioneered in Italy by Dr. Veronesi. It appears to be effective in preventing local recurrence in women with node-negative cancers that are unifocal and less than 2 centimeters in size. The advantage of intraoperative radiation is that it is a single treatment and occurs at the same time as the surgery to remove the cancer. If you are a potential candidate for intraoperative radiation based on the above criteria, you may want to inquire about entering into a clinical study using the technique. I believe that in the future intraoperative radiation given at the time of WLE will be the radiation treatment of choice for appropriate patients.

CHECKPOINTS

1. Do I need radiation?
2. What side effects should I expect, and when?
3. How long will my treatment last?
4. What are my chances of getting another cancer later in life as a result of the radiation treatment?
5. Should I have radiation before or after breast reconstruction?
6. Am I eligible for more localized radiation therapy?
7. Am I eligible for an intraoperative radiation (IORT) study?

10
· · · · · ·

Management of Side Effects

With a diagnosis of cancer, your first consideration is survival. Once you and your doctors have developed a survival plan, you can begin to consider how the treatment will alter your life. Significant progress has been made not only in the treatment of breast cancer but also in the control of the unfavorable side effects of the treatment.

Every patient will experience breast cancer and breast cancer treatment differently. You will find that physical, emotional, and spiritual aspects all play a role in how you feel and react. The extent of your side effects depends on the intensity and amount of adjuvant therapy you receive as well as your individual life experiences and your underlying sense of well-being. When diagnosed with breast cancer, most women have no symptoms. We often hear women comment on how strange it is to feel so physically normal while knowing there is a cancer in their body.

Once treatment begins, most women will feel sick, not from the cancer but from the cancer treatment. Except for the physical changes or scars, a majority, if not all, of the discomfort from cancer treatment is temporary. The purpose of this chapter is to better acquaint you with some common side effects of cancer treatment so you can work to minimize their effects and disrupt your life as little as possible. Your physicians can provide you with expectations about potential side effects and the recovery time you will most likely need for your lifestyle, responsibilities, and career.

Recovery from Surgery

✑ The standard surgery for the local control of breast cancer involves removing breast tissue. The underlying chest muscles, *pectoralis major* and *pectoralis minor*, are no longer removed as they were in the past. This advance has significantly reduced the pain and recovery time following surgery, but more important, women are spared long-term disability resulting from muscle removal. If you have a wide local excision with lymph node dissection, you will most likely have surgery and go home the same day. With removal of lymph nodes, the lymph flow from the breast is partially interrupted, and, to minimize the buildup of fluid, many surgeons will place a soft rubber tube in the wound to drain the lymph temporarily, usually for three days to a week. The drain tube from the lymph nodes empties into a closed rubber expandable vessel about the size of a handball that is on the outside of your upper body. You will usually empty the vessel daily and record the amount of fluid or lymph collected. After several days, the amount of fluid usually decreases rapidly, at which time the surgeon will remove the drain. Some surgeons do not use a drain, and if fluid builds up adjacent to the armpit wound, they drain it by inserting a needle and removing (*aspirating*) the fluid.

If lymph nodes are removed (*lymphadenectomy*), surgeons will ask that you move the involved arm as little as possible for the first few days following your surgery to allow the edges of tissue to heal and to keep lymph flow to a minimum. Once the drain is out and the wound is healing, you must begin progressive and gentle exercise of your arm to increase its range of motion in order to prevent permanent limitations that may result from scarring. Some surgeons instruct their patients on exercises, while others refer them to physical therapists who provide post-lymphadenectomy exercise instructions. It is important for you and your surgeon to discuss the option that is best for you.

Following surgery to remove lymph nodes, many women will have numbness in the armpit because nerves in the area have been damaged. Sensation often returns over several months when the nerves are healed. However, a small percentage of women will have permanent numbness in this area. For those who experience a lack of feeling, it is important to be particularly careful shaving underarm hair, and we advise patients with lost sensation in the underarm area to use an electric razor. With lymph node surgery, a small number of patients develop a clotted vein running down the inner side of the upper arm that feels like a thin cord and can restrict arm movement. If this happens, it is important to use regular heat treatments and stretching exercises to regain the full range of movement.

Side Effects of Radiation

The effect of radiation on your body is cumulative. In other words, the effect of radiation on your tissues builds up over time. The usual course of radiation is approximately twenty-five to thirty treatments. You will probably see only a few noticeable changes during the first ten or so sessions, but with continued sessions, redness and mild swelling of the skin often appear around the irradiated area. The medical technologists and staff will be watching for any unusual skin reactions and will recommend appropriate remedies to you as needed. There are creams and lotions to help ease the discomfort of skin side effects.

Most patients will experience a darkening of the radiated area that looks like a suntan. In time, as the skin heals, this usually lightens and disappears. Women have a variety of skin responses to radiation, just as people have various skin responses to sun exposure. In our own observation light-skinned women tend to have more of a visible skin reaction to radiation than those with dark skin. If you have radiation, your underlying ribs can be tender to external pressure for months to several years following treatment. Although rare, it is possible that a minor trauma can cause a rib fracture due to weakened bones following radiation. However, no special precautions need to be taken.

Many patients complain of fatigue during radiation. This can be difficult to measure, for the woman as well as for the physician. If you require chemotherapy at the same time as radiation, your fatigue may be significant. In most cases radiation is given once chemotherapy is completed. You should, therefore, be aware that your energy will be greatly diminished during your treatment and try to plan your activities accordingly.

Following breast radiation most women will have a slight skin *edema* (swelling). The easiest way to see this is at the areola, which normally appears *crinkled* but with swelling will look quite smooth. Nipple sensation and erectile ability generally remain normal. Radiation can cause the treated breast to shrink slightly. If a woman gains significant weight after radiation, it is not uncommon for the nonradiated breast to enlarge more than the one that received radiation. Also, if a woman becomes pregnant after breast radiation, the radiated breast will usually not enlarge and produce milk to the extent that the nonradiated breast will. Most of our patients who have elected to breast-feed following radiation have found that the radiated breast cannot produce a sufficient amount of milk, but the nonradiated breast functions normally.

Side Effects of Chemotherapy

As discussed in chapter 7, chemotherapy affects all rapidly dividing cells; although it destroys cancer cells, normal cells that are affected recover completely after the treatment is completed. During chemotherapy, you may experience side effects, which you should be prepared for. Nutrition during chemotherapy is extremely important because your body requires the vital nutrient *building blocks* to repair damage done to normal cells by chemotherapy. You will need a balanced diet that includes protein, which contains essential amino acids, and small amounts of fat to ensure that your cells are getting the essential fatty acids they require.

The most serious side effect of chemotherapy is the effect on the bone marrow, which can lead to decreased production of white blood cells (WBCs). This decrease in WBCs puts the body at increased risk of being unable to respond to an infection normally. Oncologists can administer *growth factors* that stimulate the bone marrow to recover more quickly after each chemotherapy treatment. Your oncologist will monitor your blood counts to determine the need for this type of supportive treatment.

In the early years of chemotherapy women were miserable with gastrointestinal distress, particularly nausea and vomiting. Today this is no longer the case due to the highly effective support drugs (5HT3 receptor antagonists) that are universally given to women receiving breast cancer chemotherapy.

Infections occurring during chemotherapy treatment will cause fever, and with any significant fever (usually higher than 101 degrees) you should notify your oncologist immediately. Most oncologists will discuss what to do in case of fever. During chemotherapy it is important to take care to prevent skin and nail infections, and if they occur, to treat them with topical antibiotics with instruction from your oncologist or chemotherapy nurse. We instruct our patients to avoid situations where they will be exposed to anyone with an active infection; otherwise there are no major restrictions about being in public places.

Chemotherapy and Menopause

Chemotherapy also affects the endocrine function of the ovaries in premenopausal women. The ovaries are the body's major source of estrogen and progesterone. They produce these hormones in a cyclical pattern in response to trigger hormones secreted by the pituitary gland. At some point in a woman's late forties or early fifties, the ovaries slow down production of these hormones, and she goes into menopause.

The process of the ovaries shutting down their hormone production takes several months to a year or more to occur. The gradual decrease in estrogen and progesterone may cause a variety of symptoms, including the cessation of menstrual periods, hot flashes or flushing, vaginal dryness, night sweats, sleep disturbance, and mood variability. A majority of premenopausal women receiving chemotherapy will have some temporary decrease in hormone production that may lead to menopausal symptoms such as hot flashes and mood changes. This means that at the very same time a woman is handling a breast cancer diagnosis, she often must deal with the changes and possible uncomfortable effects associated with menopause. This is also true for postmenopausal women on hormone replacement therapy (HRT) who suddenly must stop hormone replacement treatment as a result of the breast cancer diagnosis. In premenopausal women the ovaries will usually recover within six months of completing chemotherapy. If a woman is close to menopause at the time of chemotherapy, her ovaries may not recover and she may be put into menopause as a result of chemotherapy.

The relationship between breast cancer and estrogen is complex and controversial. The standard treatment for a newly diagnosed breast cancer patient is to stop HRT. In the past, women with breast cancer were not encouraged to begin or to resume taking HRT for the rest of their lives. This practice has changed, and treatment today is based on each woman's individual situation. You must consider the risks and benefits of HRT in relation to your specific case and discuss them with your physician(s). (Hormone replacement is discussed in further detail in chapter 15.)

Chemotherapy in the younger woman and the withdrawal of HRT in the postmenopausal patient can often produce symptoms of menopause that can be distressing and even disabling. Some of our patients turn to alternative medicines seeking relief. Certain herbs used for many years by Eastern medical practitioners contain estrogen-like substances called *phytoestrogens* (plant-based estrogens). A number of these herbs may relieve menopausal symptoms without stimulating breast cancer cells and include black cohosh, dong quai, and red clover.

Some breast cancer patients suffering from menopausal symptoms report a degree of relief results through the use of one or more of these substances, and a few report dramatic. Discuss dosage and duration of any of these supplements with your doctor.

Some women have also found that making minor dietary adjustments can result in fewer hot flashes. Soy and soy products contain an estrogen-like substance known as *genistein*. It is 1/100,000 as strong as estrogen produced by the body and may have the ability to reduce hot flashes in varying degrees for some women.

Antidepressant medications have been found to be effective in the treatment of hot flashes. The *selective serotonin reuptake inhibitors* (SSRIs) can reduce hot flashes both in number and severity. Additionally, many women note improvements in energy and quality of sleep. And very important, there are few side effects with these drugs. Venlafaxine (Effexor), paroxetine (Paxil), and fluoxetine (Prozac) have all demonstrated benefits. We usually recommend starting with Effexor at 37.5 milligrams per day. If there is no benefit after one week, we will increase the dose to 75 milligrams per day.

If antidepressants are ineffective, we often resort to the use of low-dose progesterone. The safety of low-dose progesterone in women with breast cancer has not been extensively studied, but preliminary data appear to suggest it is safe. Many oncologists use low-dose progesterone with tamoxifen, which seems to help reduce hot flashes and prevent uterine lining (endometrial) growth. Today many women are also using a natural progesterone product for these symptoms; it is made from either yams or soy and can be administered in the form of a cream. It usually requires a prescription and must be obtained from pharmacies that specialize in custom compounding; discuss this option with your oncologist. (Figure 10.1 outlines our approach to controlling menopausal symptoms.) In spite of all these options, some women on tamoxifen remain miserable. Before a patient abandons this potentially lifesaving therapy, I recommend that she add low-dose estrogen (discussed in chapter 15).

Many women experience vaginal dryness as a result of estrogen

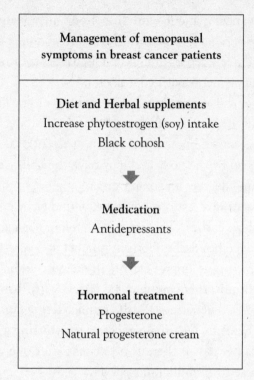

Figure 10.1

Management of menopausal symptoms in women with breast cancer

deficiency. There are a number of excellent nonhormonal vaginal mois-turizers that can offer temporary relief. Estrogen vaginal cream provides a highly effective remedy. It can be applied to the external genitalia for extra benefit. If vaginal cream is ineffective or undesirable, two good options exist. Estring is an estrogen-impregnated ring that is inserted into the vagina and slowly releases estrogen over three months. Vagi-fem is an estrogen tablet inserted into the vagina with an applicator. The tablet can be effective when used two to three times per week.

Another benefit of vaginal estrogen in addition to relieving vagi-nal dryness is a decreased risk of urinary tract infections.

Both topical estrogen and vaginal estrogen are absorbed into the bloodstream. The amount absorbed is small and should not be a concern for women with hormone receptor–negative breast cancer or women taking tamoxifen. However, women receiving an aromatase inhibitor (discussed in the previous chapter) should not use vaginal estrogen due to the risk of overcoming the *blockade* created by the AI.

Hair Loss

Certain chemotherapies cause hair loss (see chapter 7). For a majority of women, this is a devastating side effect. Chemotherapy does not cause permanent damage to the hair follicle but rather a defect in the hair protein, which causes the hair to break (Figure 10.2). Chemotherapy drugs given for breast cancer that usually cause the most significant hair loss are doxorubicin (Adriamycin), epirubicin, paclitaxel (Taxol), docetaxel (Taxotere), and oral cyclophosphamide (Cytoxan). If you are taking these drugs, you can have some loss of eyelashes, eyebrows, and pubic hair, but this is rare even with chemotherapies that cause scalp hair loss. In an attempt to reduce scalp hair loss in patients, some centers have used ice caps to freeze the scalp and

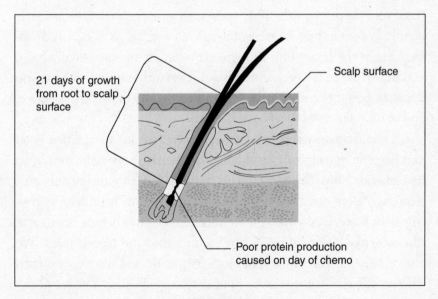

21 days of growth
from root to scalp
surface

Scalp surface

Poor protein production
caused on day of chemo

Figure 10.2
Hair follicle

prevent blood flow to hair follicles. This is only partially effective and can cause you moderate discomfort. Also, the freezing may prevent the chemotherapy from reaching the skin on the skull where, theoretically, there could be cancer cells. We do not use ice caps at our center for these reasons.

Many breast care centers have programs to help women undergoing cancer treatment with makeup, wigs, and other beauty aids. You may want to call your local cancer society for information about such programs in your area. More recently, women with chemotherapy-induced hair loss have chosen not to cover their heads. *Turning Heads*, a book published by Press on Regardless, has been inspirational to our patients. It contains many photographs of women, including the singer Melissa Etheridge, in various stages of chemotherapy-induced hair loss and recovery. You can visit its Web site at http://www.turningheadsthe book.com.

Mouth Problems

Another possible side effect of chemotherapy is the breakdown of tissues inside the mouth. This occurs because the cells that line the mouth, known as *mucous membrane*, are among the most rapidly dividing cells in the body. This lining is replaced on an almost daily basis, making these cells very vulnerable to chemotherapy (which, as you know, targets replicating cells). The lining can become thin, sensitive, and in extreme cases ulcers can develop.

To guard against this side effect, it is important to practice good oral hygiene during your treatment, while taking special care not to irritate your gums. We recommend that you have a professional teeth cleaning before starting chemotherapy and refrain from having routine dental services while you are receiving chemotherapy because of the increased risk of introducing bacteria into the bloodstream. We also advise that you brush your teeth frequently and rinse your mouth with antiseptics, but stay away from aggressive flossing. The sensitized mucous membrane is more susceptible to minor trauma and herpes infection, the danger of which can be increased with flossing. With herpes ulcers, antiviral therapy can be prescribed. If your cancer treatment results in any of these mouth problems, rinsing your mouth with a mixture of liquid Benadryl, Maalox, and viscous lidocaine may ease your discomfort (your pharmacist will prepare this mixture). Viscous lidocaine requires a prescription from your doctor. Newer agents are becoming available, so be sure to ask your medical team if mouth sores become a problem for you.

Drug Interactions

✂ Women receiving adjuvant breast cancer therapy will usually be taking a number of prescription medications as well as nonprescription drugs for symptom control and well-being. It is important to be aware of potential interactions between the different medications and chemicals you are putting in your system. For example, Benadryl interferes with tamoxifen metabolism because they both use the same activity pathway. Be sure your doctor is aware of all medications you are currently taking, and discuss any concerns about potential drug interactions with your medical team. Most pharmacies have programs that will alert you to potential adverse interactions between your current prescription drugs. Ask your pharmacist for assistance. There are also a number of online tools available that allow you to enter the name of your medication and find a list of potential interactions. Your Internet search engine is a good resource for finding these sites. We especially like the U.S. Food and Drug Administration Web site http://www.fda .gov, which provides a wealth of information about food, drugs, and other medications. Look up drugs or drug interactions at http://www .drugs.com.

There is very little literature specific to women undergoing chemotherapy that is written in plain English. One of our patients is the author of a book titled *Chemo: Secrets to Thriving: From Someone Who's*

Been There, published by NorlightsPress.com. We encourage you to read and enjoy it!

Remember that your medical team wants you to be comfortable and your cancer treatment to be as tolerable as possible. Be sure to let them know about side effects and contact your nurse specialist with any concerns.

CHECKPOINTS

1. Who is my contact person to help me manage my side effects?
2. Should I get my dental work done before I start chemotherapy or radiation?
3. What local community resources are available for me regarding my hair loss?
4. Are there any possible drug or food/drug interactions from my medications?

Breast Reconstruction

For women diagnosed with either DCIS or invasive breast cancer and who require or desire mastectomy, there has been tremendous progress in the area of breast reconstruction over the last few years. Today the breast cancer surgeon and the plastic surgeon (reconstruction surgeon) work together to form a presurgery plan that results in a far superior outcome compared to earlier attempts at breast reconstruction. The old method involved the plastic surgeon seeing the woman after her mastectomy and attempting to create a reconstruction on a chest wall left with a large scar and limited skin.

In my opinion the present superior and often spectacular results are due to four major developments.

1. Preoperative planning with the breast cancer surgeons and plastic surgeon working together.
2. The emergence of plastic surgeons who specialize in breast reconstruction and who are passionate about what they do.
3. New materials and devices that aid in the reconstruction process.
4. New surgical techniques that often involve skin and even nipple preservation.

The cosmetic result achieved after immediate reconstruction with a skin- and nipple-sparing procedure can be better than that following wide local excision plus radiation. This option eliminates the need for annual surveillance for local recurrence and the five to six weeks required for radiation therapy. At our centers there is an increasing trend in women choosing mastectomy with reconstruction over breast conservation with radiation. If you and your team are considering mastectomy, it is critical that you consult with the plastic surgeon *prior to* your cancer surgery. These surgical techniques are relatively new and require a high level of coordination and technical skill from the breast surgeon and the plastic surgeon. Don't be afraid to ask the surgical team about the extent of their experience in this type of reconstruction. The best results are achieved when the surgeon has a passion and commitment for the best outcome possible. You may want to ask if it is possible to talk on the phone or in person with women who have had the procedure performed by your surgeon.

There are two basic methods of breast reconstruction. The first involves the use of an *expander* which is placed beneath the chest muscle (*pectoralis muscle*) at the time of the mastectomy or as a second procedure depending on patient preference. The chest muscle and skin are then expanded, creating a space that serves as the location for the permanent saline or silicone implant that will be inserted during a second procedure (Figure 11.1). This is the most commonly performed procedure for breast reconstruction in the United States in part because it allows women the most rapid return to their normal activity.

The second method of breast reconstruction, called a *flap reconstruction*, involves bringing skin and fat to the breast from another area of the body. The usual sites of donor tissue are the patient's tummy (abdomen) or the back. This surgery is more complex and results in an additional scar and site of healing. The advantage of this reconstruction procedure is that it uses a woman's own tissue, eliminating the need for a foreign silicone implant.

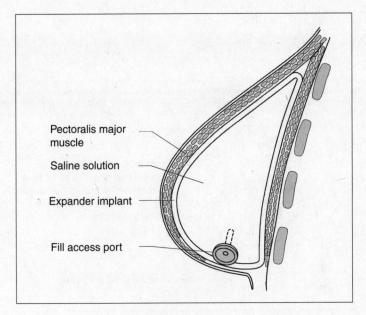

Pectoralis major
muscle

Saline solution

Expander implant

Fill access port

Figure 11.1
Breast reconstruction expander

There are two techniques for flap reconstruction. The first involves transferring tissue without disrupting the blood supply (Figure 11.2). This is called a *pedicle transfer* and involves freeing tissue in the abdomen and transferring it to the reconstruction site through a tunnel created by the surgeon beneath the skin. The purpose for moving the abdominal tissue through the tunnel is so that it will retain its intact blood supply with little risk of tissue *necrosis*. The procedure from the abdomen is called a TRAM (Transverse Rectus Abdominis Myocutaneous). A similar procedure can be done from the back using the *latissimus muscle*. The reason that muscle must be transferred with the overlying fat is that they share a blood supply.

The second technique involves removing fat and tissue from the body along with their blood vessels, transferring these to the new site, and reconnecting the blood vessels to existing blood vessels at the new site. Termed a *free tissue transfer* (*free TRAM* or *DIEP flap*), this

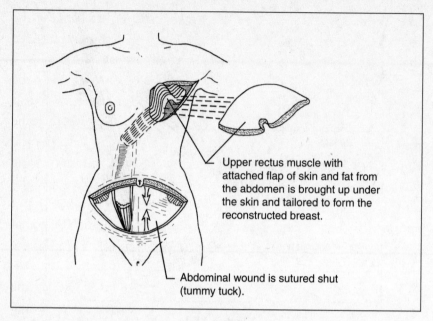

Upper rectus muscle with attached flap of skin and fat from the abdomen is brought up under the skin and tailored to form the reconstructed breast.

Abdominal wound is sutured shut (tummy tuck).

Figure 11.2

Breast reconstruction—tissue transfer

procedure is usually done using the patient's abdominal tissue, and in many cases little muscle needs to be transferred. Special microvascular techniques are required, and the plastic surgeon should specialize in the procedure. This procedure is complex, and includes risk of tissue necrosis. It also requires a number of days in the hospital. The advantage over the TRAM procedure is that there is less deformity from the procedure and much less muscle is removed from the abdomen.

There are advantages and disadvantages with both reconstruction methods, and it is important to discuss these with your physician. Decisions about the type of reconstruction are based upon the cancer operation itself (the extent of skin removed and the location of scars) and the amount of fat available to be transferred.

A majority of women at our centers undergo expander-type reconstruction. On the whole it is a less complex procedure, and when the surgeons can preserve skin and even the nipple, the result is excellent.

In the past, there has been controversy about the use of silicone at the reconstruction site. Based on extensive studies, the FDA has concluded that the current generation of silicone implants are safe and durable.

A potential cosmetic problem of expander reconstruction is the coverage of tissue and skin over the silicone implant. If the coverage is too thin, there can be problems with healing (*flap necrosis*), or the results can be less than natural, with visible *ripples*. The key is for the cancer surgeon to make the skin flaps thick enough with underlying subcutaneous fat to cover the implant without leaving breast glandular tissue. Leaving glandular breast tissue behind increases the risk of a future cancer or a recurrence, while a layer of subcutaneous fat that is too thin can result in a less than acceptable outcome. This is where the experience and skill of the breast surgeon are critical.

Plastic surgeons today often combine additional procedures during reconstruction to optimize the results of implant reconstruction. Many surgeons utilize sheets of inert *collagen* (AlloDerm) to add more protective coverage over implants while obtaining a more cosmetically appealing result. Some surgeons will even combine the back flap procedure (latissimus) with expander reconstruction to allow better coverage and more volume. The reconstruction plan is tailored to the individual patient's goals and needs.

The new era of breast reconstruction has given women who require or desire mastectomy(ies) excellent cosmetic results. Some women who are prime candidates for WLE with radiation are choosing mastectomy(ies) instead to reduce the risk of future breast cancers and to alleviate continued surveillance and potential biopsies.

For those women who decide to have breast preservation with WLE, surgeons are now using reconstructive techniques at the time of the surgery, with improved cosmetic results. These techniques, termed *oncoplastic surgery*, involve special approaches to remove the cancer and rearrange the remaining breast tissue to give superior cosmetic outcomes. This often involves some surgery to the unaffected breast as well to provide balance and symmetry.

In summary, we have come a very long way since the radical

mastectomy. Our goal now, as it was then, is to achieve local control and remove all cancer from the breast. With spectacular new surgical techniques, women can go on with their lives after breast cancer surgery feeling whole and self-confident and without compromising their chance to be cured. This requires that you understand and discuss these aspects of your care with the surgical members of your treatment team.

CHECKPOINTS

1. Am I a candidate for immediate reconstruction?
2. Am I better suited for the expander-type reconstruction rather than tissue-transfer reconstruction?
3. Am I a candidate for nipple preservation?
4. Should I see a plastic surgeon? Does my breast surgeon work with an experienced plastic surgeon who specializes in breast reconstruction?
5. Should I consider bilateral mastectomy?

Clinical Research Trials

Progress in the treatment and cure of breast cancer has been painfully slow. Fortunately, due to accelerated research programs and development of new treatment options, we appear to be entering a new era in cancer diagnosis and treatment. Funding from private philanthropies, the government, and private industry sponsors has driven all areas of breast cancer research, and the results are very promising. Understanding that breast cancer is due to a number of genetic mutations, scientists have refocused their efforts on finding ways to target therapy that can reverse or eliminate malignant cells within the body. This type of therapy is very different from the toxic chemotherapies that were the mainstay of adjuvant therapy in the past.

In the last several years we have seen a new targeted therapy, trastuzumab (Herceptin), become the standard treatment for *Her2-overexpressing* breast cancer. Lapatinib (Tykerb) is moving quickly through the testing process and will soon be used in early *Her2-positive cancers*. Bevacizumab (Avastin), the *antiangiogenesis* drug previously approved for the treatment of colon cancer, is rapidly proceeding through clinical trials for breast cancer. All of these drugs, as well as many more in the research pipeline, are specifically targeted at the mutated cancer cell, leaving the normal healthy cells alone.

Besides drug development, clinical research involves the development of new therapeutic and diagnostic procedures. These new technologies are expensive and must be proven to be safe, helpful, and cost-effective. Sentinel lymph node sampling, MRI and PET scanning are a few examples of procedures that are now a part of standard breast cancer care. Treatment changes can only occur after physicians and their patients are convinced that a new treatment or procedure is superior to what is already available. This process of demonstrating whether a new therapy is better than the previous standard therapy requires that women volunteer to participate in the testing of new medications and treatment options. Such projects are known as *clinical research trials.*

Research trials must be conducted in an unbiased, fair way so that the results are reliable. This requires that women be randomly entered into different treatment groups. Eventually, the outcomes of each group in the trial are compared against one another. For example, data drawn from past clinical trials have provided the following important results:

- Less surgery plus radiation is as effective as mastectomy in Stage 1 or 2 breast cancer.
- Giving chemotherapy to women with local breast cancer prevents the development of metastatic disease.
- Tamoxifen increases the cure rate in women with hormone-positive breast cancer.

The randomized clinical trial eliminates physician and investigator bias, an important issue in trials comparing new therapy with standard therapies. The major breast cancer research group in this country and possibly the world is the National Surgical Adjuvant Breast and Bowel Project, known as the NSABP. This group includes surgeons and radiation and medical oncologists from all parts of North America and has conducted more than thirty-five randomized trials in breast cancer over the past thirty-five years. The NSABP is responsible for the majority of progress made in breast cancer treatment.

Patients who have been willing to participate in clinical research studies have made a significant contribution to medical progress for all of society. Each trial tests a new hypothesis, or theory, and the results then become the knowledge base for the next clinical trial. In order to show significant differences in therapy, several thousand women are needed as volunteers in each trial. The volunteers realize that they may be getting the established or the experimental treatment, and they will most likely not be told which they are receiving. They bravely participate with this degree of uncertainty. The pioneer women were those who agreed to go into clinical trials comparing mastectomy to WLE or chemotherapy versus a placebo. These women didn't know if one treatment was more or less effective than the other, but they agreed to help answer the research question: *which of these therapies is optimal?*

Today research trials compare the standard of practice, or current state of the art in breast cancer treatment, to what might *potentially* be better. The difference in treatment plans involves the sequencing of different therapies or the addition of a new drug. There are many opportunities to participate in clinical research trials in which you would receive state-of-the-art care. The National Cancer Institute (NCI) sponsors researchers around the United States and world including the NSABP, Southwest Oncology Group (SWOG), and the Cancer and Leukemia-Group B (CALGB). In order to participate in a clinical study, you must be willing to be randomly assigned to a treatment group. You will be asked to carefully read and sign a detailed informed consent document that explains the research purpose and procedures and the risks and benefits involved with participation. Many community-based oncologists participate in cooperative trials sponsored by the National Cancer Institute (NCI), and if you are interested, you should discuss this option with your physician and treatment team.

Information about clinical trials is available from NCI's Cancer Information Service at 1-800-4-CANCER and in the NCI booklet *Taking Part in Cancer Treatment Research Studies*, which can be found at http://www.cancer.gov/publications. This booklet describes how research studies are carried out and explains possible risks and benefits. Further information about clinical trials is available on the NCI Web site: http://www.cancer.gov/clinicaltrials. The Web site offers detailed information about specific ongoing studies by linking to PDQ, NCI's comprehensive cancer information database.

In addition to clinical research trials, there are a number of small research projects available called *pilot studies*. These small studies are often designed to explore novel and cutting-edge ideas or therapies and are usually not randomized. They are often underwritten by pharmaceutical companies or entrepreneurial companies, and many are conducted at teaching hospitals and universities. As in all research, safeguards are in place to protect participating individuals to the greatest extent possible. Pilot study protocols are usually designed for women with advanced disease who are willing to place themselves at some increased risk because of limited available alternatives at a late stage of disease.

Human clinical trials are separated into three phases depending on the questions that each one is attempting to answer. *Phase I* testing is designed to determine if a promising treatment has acceptable tolerance in patients and at what dosage significant side effects appear. Once an agent, drug, or treatment has been proven safe, *Phase II* testing begins. This second phase quantifies the objective response rate (measures the reduction in cancer) resulting from use of the agent, drug, or treatment being tested. In women with breast cancer, both Phase I and Phase II testing are performed on patients with metastatic disease. *Phase III* testing compares the current, standard treatment to a promising new treatment that has completed Phase I and Phase II testing. Most of the trials for women with newly diagnosed breast cancer are Phase III trials. The clinical trial process of testing new therapy requires an orderly process that ensures safety and accuracy. For many of us, physicians and patients, this process seems too slow. To speed things up, the world breast cancer research community must collaborate and coordinate to eliminate duplication of clinical trial research. As more women enter trials, progress toward results will continue to increase.

We are very interested in testing promising new therapies in the *neoadjuvant* (preoperative) setting using the primary cancer's response to a new drug or treatment. If the primary cancer disappears completely, we know there is a high probability of cure. Research of this type allows for much faster progress because we do not have to wait years for a systemic relapse to determine differences between treatment groups.

Another type of research trial is the large, *epidemiologic* (population-based) research study. These types of studies are not clinical trials. Instead, they examine the cause, distribution, and control of disease (in our case breast cancer) in populations. Groups or populations of people are examined to identify who is affected by a particular disorder, changes in incidence and mortality over time are studied, and associated risk factors are proposed. Epidemiologic data are used to recognize those groups at high risk for a disease and recommend preventive measures that impact on public health policies and future clinical trials research. This type of research often relies on lengthy surveys, health, and family history questionnaires, and sometimes the collection of biospecimen samples such as blood or saliva or tumor tissue. Because epidemiologic studies are not clinical trials, they do not provide medical care or treatment, and you will probably not receive personalized results from any testing done using the information or samples you provide. Some of the things that breast cancer epidemiologists seek to identify include: (1) women within a population who may be at risk for developing breast cancer; (2) the geographic location where breast cancer risk is highest; (3) when it will likely occur and trends over time; (4) exposures that breast cancer patients have in common; (5) how much the risk is increased through exposure; and (6) how many breast cancer cases could be prevented through elimination of the exposure.

Our advice is to ask your doctors if you are eligible for any research trials. Also inquire as to whether they participate as investigators in any studies or if there is a research center participating with one of the cooperative groups near you. Your ability to participate may depend upon the type of health care delivery system you are in, so you will want to talk to your insurance company or HMO representative as well. In general, the next several years should prove very exciting in the field of breast cancer clinical research because enormous financial and scientific resources are being devoted to determining the cause of breast cancer and development of new agents aimed at prevention and cure.

CHECKPOINTS

1. Am I eligible for a current, nationally sponsored clinical research trial?
2. Do my doctors participate in clinical research? If yes, what type?
3. What cooperative group protocol am I eligible for?
4. Is the therapy my doctors are recommending for me similar to any clinical research trial or pilot study?

Understanding Genetic Risk

CREATING A FAMILY HEALTH PEDIGREE

All cancer is *genetic*. That is to say, in order for a normal cell to change into a cancer cell, a genetic mistake must occur. Genetic mistakes, or *mutations*, occur quite frequently in the human body, and specialized mechanisms are in place to repair these errors. Many mutations are of little consequence and simply vanish; however, if a mistake occurs in a critical location within a cell, cancer can result. Cancer usually requires several separate events to occur over time; a single mistake or mutation does not usually lead to a cancer. For many women breast cancer is the result of a number of random genetic mistakes. This may explain the presence of certain *precancerous* conditions, such as *atypical lobular neoplasia*, often found in biopsies. This condition may indicate that cells have experienced first or even second mutations but have not yet gone on to become cancer. Once cells are "primed," it takes only the final mutation to develop into cancer. On the other hand, some women are predisposed to breast cancer because they have *inherited* one or more genetic mutations. From research we know that there is at least one inherited defective gene that interferes with the process of repairing genetic mistakes. In this case, a mutation that would normally be repaired is not. This can lead to a cascade of unfortunate gene events that will ultimately result in a breast cancer.

Our knowledge of human genetics seems to increase daily. Internationally, researchers are attempting to unravel the genetic message contained within each cell. With a better understanding of the human genome, gene therapy will soon be available for use as a preventive strategy for those women who have a predisposing genetic abnormality. This may eventually have further application for all women with breast cancer.

Understanding the genetics of cancer will most likely increase tremendously over the next several years. Here are some general principles about cancer genetics that are known at this time.

- Genes produce protein messengers that stimulate uncontrolled cell growth *or* suppress the protein function necessary to stop cells from growing out of control.
- Defective genes that produce either type of protein messenger in abnormal quantities or with defects can lead to cancer.

There are three types of gene defects that appear to lead to cancer:

1. *Oncogene production.* This type of mutation leads to the production of proteins that *promote* the malignant transformation of the cell. An example is the Her-2 oncogene.
2. *Tumor-suppressor gene defect.* The tumor-suppressor gene functions normally to produce proteins that protect cells against malignant change. When the gene produces defective or missing proteins, cancer can occur.
3. *Mutator genes.* These abnormal genes accelerate the production of oncogenes, or defective tumor-suppressor genes.

About 90 percent of breast cancer appears to be the *sporadic type*, which means the cancer occurs randomly without an underlying defect in the patient's cells. However, about 10 percent of women with breast cancer have inherited a genetic mutation that has caused them to be predisposed to this disease. There are several hundred cancer genetic syndromes but only a few syndromes in which we see breast cancer commonly occur. Each person is born with two copies of every gene, one inherited from their mother and one from their father. When a condition is inherited in a *dominant* fashion (one from either mother or father), it only takes one mistake (mutation) in one of the genes to cause a susceptibility (*autosomal*). Most of the breast cancer syndromes are inherited in an autosomal dominant fashion. When a condition is *recessive, both copies* (one from both mother and father) in an inherited pair must be mutated.

In the early 1990s a groundbreaking discovery identified the first gene that could lead to increased risk of breast cancer. This gene, termed the *1st BReast CAncer gene* (BRCA1), belongs to a class of genes known as *tumor-suppressor genes* because they prevent cells from growing and dividing too rapidly or in an uncontrolled way. The BRCA1 gene inhibits the growth of cells that line the milk ducts of the breast and provides instructions for making a protein that is directly involved in the repair of damaged DNA. By repairing DNA, BRCA1 and other proteins play an important role in maintaining the stability of a cell's genetic information. When a mutation occurs in the BRCA1 gene the result is increased risk of breast cancer.

Researchers have followed hundreds of families that carry the BRCA1 autosomal dominant mutation. Approximately 60 to 80 percent of women with this mutation will go on to develop breast cancer. Moreover, breast epithelial cells are not the only susceptible cells. Between 25 and 44 percent of women with BRCA1 mutation will develop ovarian cancer. Since this is an autosomal defect, the children of an affected person will have a 50 percent chance of inheriting the defective gene. It is a common misconception that breast cancer risk cannot be inherited from the father. Fully 50 percent of hereditary breast cancer is inherited through the paternal side. Men with the defect can develop breast cancer, but this risk is fairly low. They do, however, have a significantly higher incidence of early onset prostate cancer.

Soon after the discovery of BRCA1, scientists discovered another gene that can contribute to an increase in breast cancer susceptibility when a mutation is present. This gene, termed the *2nd BReast CAncer gene (BRCA2)*, is found on chromosome 13. The incidence of BRCA2 mutations appears to be slightly less than that of BRCA1 mutations. BRCA2 is also inherited in an autosomal dominant fashion. The lifetime risk of breast cancer with a BRCA2 mutation is greater than 50 percent. Initially it was believed that the presence of the BRCA2 gene defect did not appear to increase the risk for ovarian cancer. However, it is now clear that these mutations do increase the risk of ovarian cancer, perhaps by as much as 20 to 25 percent. This is not as high as with the mutations in BRCA1, but significant nonetheless. It also appears that men with the defect have an increased incidence of breast cancer. (The differences between BRCA1 and BRCA2 are listed in Table 13.1.)

While we wait for more breakthroughs, researchers and physicians continue to gather information about breast cancer by studying breast cancer tumor tissue and patient blood samples. Additional research is now ongoing with animals that have been specifically bred to have the breast cancer characteristics of interest to their research. Commercial genetic testing for breast cancer genes is available as well. Armed with this patient information, the medical community can counsel women on strategies for surveillance, prevention, and risk-reduction interventions.

If we are going to do genetic testing and find out information about women, we need to be sure that we have the appropriate mechanisms in place and an action plan to deal with the situation and reduce anxiety.

One area of particular concern for women with newly diagnosed breast cancer is the possible risk of cancer to their children, especially daughters. *Every* woman and/or family who pursues genetic testing should seek professional genetic counseling from a physician or a genetic counselor before proceeding with testing. During the genetic counseling session a number of issues will be addressed to help you to clearly understand the meaning of the test results and available treatment options. The important questions the physician or counselor will

BRCA1 Mutation—women
- Approximately 0.3% (1 in 333) of women diagnosed with breast cancer have a BRCA1 mutation
- Average 65 percent lifetime risk for developing breast cancer
- 40 to 60 percent lifetime risk for second breast cancer (not reappearance of first tumor)
- Average 39 percent lifetime risk for ovarian cancer
- Increased risk for other cancer types such as cervical cancer, uterine cancer, pancreas cancer, and colon cancer

BRCA1 Mutation—men
- Increased risk for developing cancer such as breast cancer, early onset prostate cancer, pancreas cancer, and testicular cancer (however in men, breast cancer, prostate cancer, and pancreas cancer appear to be more strongly associated with BRCA2 mutation)

BRCA2 Mutation—women
- Average 65 percent lifetime risk for breast cancer
- Approximately 0.12% of women (1 in 833) with breast cancer will have a BRCA2 mutation
- Average 11 percent lifetime risk for ovarian cancer
- Increased risk for other cancer types, such as pancreas cancer, stomach cancer, gall bladder cancer, bile duct cancer, and melanoma

BRCA2 Mutation—men
- Increased risk for developing breast cancer, pancreas cancer, and prostate cancer

Table 13.1

Risks associated with BRCA1 and BRCA2 mutations in women and men

help you answer include: If you were to obtain genetic information about yourself, would you do anything differently based on those results? Is this information that you really want or need to have? Do you have family members who might be affected by the results, and do they really want to know the results?

In most cases, when evaluating women for BRCA1 or BRCA2

mutation, we examine the family tree, or *pedigree*, looking for all cases of breast and other cancers. If there are very few cases of breast cancer in the family, the woman most likely does not have a genetic mutation. On the other hand, if about half the women on either side of the family have breast cancer, the patient may carry the BRCA1 or BRCA2 gene mutation. This is, of course, dependent on the size and number of women in the family; thus reviewing your complete family history with your physician and/or with a genetic counselor can provide you with a more accurate estimation of risk. In general, the risk of carrying a BRCA mutation tends to be higher in: (1) individuals diagnosed with breast cancer before the age of fifty, (2) women whose family history includes relatives diagnosed with premenopausal breast or ovarian cancer, and/or (3) women of Ashkenazi Jewish ancestry.

It is helpful to create a family tree for your physicians and for your own records to help determine if such a pattern exists and if your doctors should be concerned about any other type of inherited breast cancer risk. In the development of the family tree, you will be called the *index case* (usually identified by an arrow), and you will include your two parents and two sets of grandparents. Then fill in information on your aunts, uncles, cousins, and siblings, listing any diseases, cancers, and the cause of death for all of those who are deceased. (Figure 13.1 presents an example of a family health history formatted as a picture pedigree. Table 13.2 presents the same health information in table format.) If you are interested in creating your own unique family health pedigree, you can choose from a number of different Web sites on the Internet that will help you do so. The U.S. Department of Health and Human Services family history Web site was used to develop our sample family health pedigree: https://familyhistory.hhs .gov. On this site you can enter and update family health information, share your pedigree with extended family members online, and save or print your family history documents. Once you have entered your family history information on the Web site, the program will produce a spreadsheet and family pedigree (Figure 13.1). For record keeping,

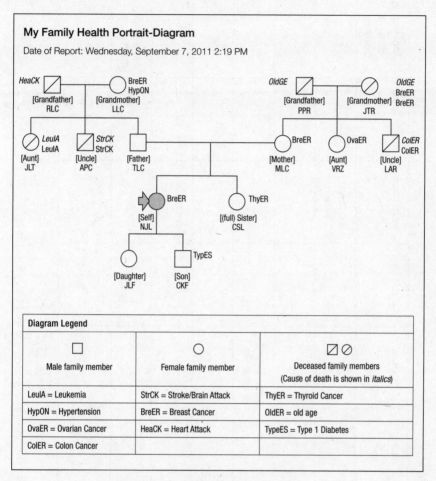

Figure 13.1

Sample family health picture pedigree for cancer risk

include the initials of relatives along with each one's current age or age at death, the date and cause of death where relevant, and any major diseases.

Many women are understandably concerned about the risk of developing a second breast cancer. If your cancer is the *ductal* type, if you have no hereditary breast cancer pattern in your family, and if you have no associated lobular neoplasia, your risk for recurrence is close

My Family Health Portrait—Table

Date of Report: Wednesday, September 7, 2011 2:19 PM

	Still living?	Heart Disease	Stroke	Diabetes	Colon Cancer	Breast Cancer	Ovarian Cancer	Additional Diseases or Conditions
NJL (Self)	Yes					Breast Cancer (40–49 years)		
JLF (Daughter)	Yes							
CKF (Son)	Yes			Type 1 Diabetes (in Childhood)				
TLC (Father)	Yes							
MLC (Mother)	Yes					Breast Cancer (50–59 years)		
CSL (full Sister)	Yes							Thyroid Cancer (40–49 years)
RLC (Paternal Grandfather)	No, Heart Attack (60 years and older)	Heart Attack (null)						

Table 13.2

Sample family health information table for cancer risk

Risk category	Per-year risk (%)	Lifetime Risk (%)
Lobular neoplasia	0.5–1.0	12–20
Ductal or lobular cancer with associated lobular neoplasia	1.0–2.0	30
BRCA 1 or BRCA 2 mutation	5–6	>50

Table 13.3

Breast cancer incidence for *high-risk women*

to the average woman's risk (no greater than a 12 percent lifetime risk or less than 0.5 percent per year). However, if you have a *lobular* breast cancer or associated lobular neoplasia (*LCIS* or *atypical lobular hyperplasia*), your risk of developing a second breast cancer is higher, approximately 1 to 2 percent per year or a 30 percent lifetime risk. Having a BRCA1 mutation is associated with a 25 to 30 percent risk of a second breast cancer within five years of the first diagnosis, and it is assumed that mutations in BRCA2 are associated with comparable risks. In addition, mutations in either BRCA1 or BRCA2 make it ten times more likely that a woman with breast cancer will later develop cancer of the ovary. Table 13.3 summarizes your risk. From this table you can determine what decisions need to be made regarding further preventive measures to avoid a breast cancer recurrence.

Only one U.S. laboratory, Myriad Genetics, offers full analysis for BRCA1 and BRCA2 outside of specific research projects. The test performed is designed to find any of the hundreds of different mutations in these genes that have been identified. (The Web sites and phone number of Myriad Genetics are provided in the Resources section of this book.)

Clearly, the ability to identify women at increased risk for both ovarian and breast cancer is helpful in our surveillance and prevention of these diseases. A government panel of experts has recommended that women with BRCA1 or BRCA2 gene mutations be monitored for breast and ovarian cancer beginning around the age of twenty-five. This would include monthly breast self-examination, annual or semi-annual clinician evaluation, and annual breast imaging. For women under age thirty, MRI is the procedure of choice because there is no radiation exposure and the MRI images are not affected by breast density, which decreases with age.

It is recommended that women who are positive for one of the genetic mutations undergo annual breast MRI screening. In addition, there is evidence that the drug tamoxifen (chapter 8) may help to reduce the risk of breast cancer in women with the BRCA2 gene mutation. Women with hereditary risk often choose surgical removal of the breasts (*prophylactic mastectomy*), which has been shown to reduce the risk of breast cancer by greater than 90 percent. With the tremendous progress in breast reconstruction at the time of mastectomies, more women are undergoing preventive surgery.

Women with either BRCA1 or BRCA2 mutation may also choose to be screened and monitored for ovarian cancer. Screening methods include abdominal ultrasound using an intravaginal probe and a blood test called *CA-125*, although neither of these methods is as effective as we would hope in identifying early-stage ovarian cancer. There are, however, treatments that may reduce the risk of ovarian cancer. For example, a recent study demonstrated that women with a gene mutation who took birth control pills for approximately five years were far less likely to develop ovarian cancer. Finally, surgical removal of the ovaries might be considered, usually after age thirty-five or after childbearing is completed. Like prophylactic mastectomy, this procedure greatly reduces but does not entirely eliminate the risk of ovarian cancer.

Since a large number of human diseases have a genetic basis, we are certain to see major medical breakthroughs in the near future. Breast cancer will be among the diseases that will benefit from genetic research, and we are cautiously optimistic that there will soon be a *cure*.

CHECKPOINTS

1. Have I completed a family health history and developed a pedigree? Have I discussed my family health history with my doctor?
2. If I assess my family history and determine that a BRCA1 or BRCA2 mutation is a possibility, what course of action is recommended?
3. What is my risk of a second breast cancer? Was there any lobular neoplasia in my biopsy?
4. What is the course of action recommended if my family history determines that I may be at risk for BRCA1 or BRCA2 mutation?

14
· · · · · ·
❧

Nutrition, Supplements, and Herbal Remedies

In this chapter we discuss the role that nutrition plays in cancer risk reduction and cancer treatment. Quite popular now on the Internet, television, and in different publications are testimonials suggesting that breast cancer can be prevented, and even cured, with dietary and lifestyle changes. This approach has a certain appeal to us because it is simple, empowering, and provides us with guidelines that we can understand and follow. While there is no special diet that will prevent the development of breast cancer and no food or meal plan that is a breast cancer cure, there are a variety of foods that can help you to be as healthy as possible, enhance your immune system, and keep the risk of primary diagnosis or recurrence *as low as possible*.

Food and nutrition are an essential part of your breast cancer treatment plan. In order to support and promote the growth of healthy cells, nutrients found in a healthy diet will help you to retain your energy and strength. After your breast cancer treatment has finished, a healthy diet will also help your body heal and may even protect it in the future. By eating well during your cancer treatment you will: (1) restore your strength and energy levels, (2) find it easier to tolerate the side effects from treatment, (3) reduce your risk of infection, (4) heal and recover faster, and (5) feel better!

Cancer and cancer treatments do have an impact on nutrition. Prior to a cancer diagnosis, most women do not have a problem getting all of the nutrients that their bodies need. But after treatments begin, this may be more difficult, especially if patients experience unpleasant side effects or generally "just don't feel well." Most treatment plans involve at least one of the following: surgery, radiation therapy, chemotherapy, hormonal therapy—or a combination of these treatments. While designed to kill cancer cells, these therapies can also destroy some healthy cells, resulting in side effects that impact on your ability to eat, including loss of appetite, changes in taste or smell, weight loss, fatigue, or a sore mouth or throat.

During cancer treatment we recommend that you obtain the majority of your nutrients from a healthy diet that includes a variety of foods. If you find that you cannot get enough calories at mealtime, you may want to ask your oncologist about including a nutritional supplement drink that contains a variety of vitamins and minerals. The nutrients that you need to help your body fight cancer include protein, carbohydrates, fat, water, and vitamins and minerals.

Eating Right during Treatment

Protein

It is generally recommended that breast cancer patients include a diet that is high in protein to provide the building blocks that a body needs. Protein is necessary to repair body tissue and help the immune system to stay strong; patients who do not consume enough protein may have lower resistance to infection and may take longer to recover. Good sources of high-protein foods include low and nonfat milk products, eggs, lean meats, fish, and poultry, as well as dried beans, peas, lentils, nuts, and soy foods. (For the relationship between soy and breast cancer, see the final section of this chapter.) Eating a variety of protein foods, including at least two to three servings of seafood per week, will improve nutrient intake and health benefits. However, choosing protein foods that are high in saturated fat and cholesterol may not contribute to a healthy diet.

Quick tips about protein:

- Lean meat, fish, poultry, dry beans and peas, eggs, nuts, and seeds supply many nutrients including B vitamins (niacin, thiamin, riboflavin, and B6), vitamin E, iron, zinc, and magnesium.
- Proteins act as building blocks for muscles, cartilage, skin, and blood. They also play an important role with enzymes, hormones, and vitamins.
- Choose fat-free or low-fat dairy products. Dairy products provide calcium, potassium, vitamin D, and protein, nutrients that are essential for health and body maintenance. The intake of dairy foods is linked to improved bone health, reduced risk of osteoporosis, reduced risk of cardiovascular disease and type 2 diabetes, and with reducing blood pressure.
- When choosing protein foods, *go lean* and *keep it lean*. Choose the leanest cuts of beef, pork, ground beef, chicken, and turkey. Trim away visible fat and remove the skin from chicken before cooking. Broil, grill, roast, poach, or boil meat, poultry, or fish instead of frying.
- Prepare beans and peas without added fat and don't use high-fat sauces or gravies.
- Choose seafood at least twice a week as it is high in omega-3 fatty acids. Omega-3 fatty acids (EPA and DHA) are involved in many body activities, especially immune system responses.
- Nuts and seeds are high in calories, so eat them in small portions and use them to replace other protein foods, like meat or poultry, rather than adding them to what you already eat.

Carbohydrates

Carbohydrates are the major source of energy for your body, and they are necessary for physical activity and proper organ function. Good sources of carbohydrates also supply to the body's cells needed vitamins and minerals, fiber, and *phytochemicals* (chemicals found in plants). Fruits, vegetables, grains and pasta, cereals, crackers, dried beans, peas, and lentils are all good sources of carbohydrate, and many are also good sources of dietary fiber, which your digestive system needs to stay healthy.

Quick tips about carbohydrates:

- *Whole grains*—wheat, oats, corn, and rye, along with lesser-known grains such as barley, spelt, groats, wheat berries, millet, and flax-seed. These grains and the foods made from them contain naturally occurring nutrients in the *grain seed* and include several B vitamins (thiamin, riboflavin, niacin, and folate) and minerals (iron, magnesium, and selenium). Look for whole grains in cereals, breads, flours, and crackers, and check labels for the words *whole* or *whole grain*. Some whole grains can be prepared and used as a side dish or meal.

- *Fiber*—the part of the plant that the body is unable to digest. Fiber helps to move food waste through the digestive tract and out of the body quickly. Some anticancer drugs and other drugs such as pain medications may cause constipation. This problem can also occur if your diet does not include enough fiber or fluid or if you haven't been getting enough exercise. Be sure to include lots of whole grains in your daily menu. Great sources of fiber include fruits and vegetables, whole grains, and all types of beans. Choose whole fruits whenever you can as these contain a lot more fiber and far fewer calories than fruit juice. In addition to fiber, beans are a good source of protein; they are inexpensive, and they contribute more nutrients. Fruits and vegetables are important sources of potassium, folate, and also vitamins A and C which help to protect cells from damage.

- *Sweeteners*—white or brown sugar, honey, or molasses. These carbohydrates are high in calories and don't offer any other benefits such as vitamins, minerals, or fiber. When selecting good sources of carbohydrates, it is best to choose whole grains, fruits, and vegetables.

- *Phytochemicals*—compounds produced by plants that are thought to provide health-protecting benefits. Found in fruits, vegetables, grains, beans, and other plants, phytochemicals may help to protect cells from damage.

In addition to maintaining a healthy diet during your breast cancer treatment, it is important to achieve optimal health after your treatments are completed. Carbohydrates play a significant role in this regard. Consuming whole grains can help to reduce your risk of heart disease, high blood pressure, obesity, and diabetes. B vitamins play a role in metabolism and are essential for a healthy nervous system. Folate helps the body form red blood cells, and iron is used to help cells carry oxygen in the blood. Eat foods high in vitamin C, along with whole grain products, to increase iron absorption from these foods. Vitamin C also helps with wound and cut healing and keeps teeth and gums healthy.

Eating potassium-rich foods is important to maintain healthy blood pressure, and it may also reduce the risk of kidney stones and help to decrease bone loss. Vitamin A keeps eyes and skin healthy while protecting against infection. Last, magnesium found in whole-grain foods helps to build bones and release energy from muscles, while selenium is important for a healthy immune system.

Be sure to wash fresh fruits and vegetables carefully as cancer treatments can compromise your immune system.

Fats and Oils

You do need some fat in your diet, just not very much. Fats play an important role in nutrition and serve as a rich source of energy for the body. However, it's a good idea to keep your fat intake low. Fat should comprise no more than 10 to 20 percent of your total daily calories. Fats and oils are made up of fatty acids and are used to store energy, insulate body organs and tissues, and transport vitamins through the blood. As you already know, some fats are better for you than others.

The three main types of fat are:

- *Monounsaturated fats*. These *good fats* are found mainly in vegetable oils, like canola, olive, and peanut oil, that can help to lower your LDL cholesterol. This type of fat is liquid at room temperature.

- *Polyunsaturated fats*. Sources of these *good fats* include vegetable oils like safflower, sunflower, corn, flaxseed, and canola oils. They are also the main type of fat found in seafood (*omega-3 fatty acids*). Certain polyunsaturated fatty acids, called *essential fatty acids*, are needed by the body to build cells and make hormones. Because the human body cannot make essential fatty acids, they can only come from the foods that you eat. Research has shown that one of the essential fatty acids, omega-3, is especially important in immune system response and can help reduce the risk of heart disease. Research to date has not shown an association between omega-3 fatty acids and breast cancer risk.

- *Saturated fats*. These so-called *bad fats* raise blood cholesterol levels. They are found mainly in animal sources like meat and poultry, whole milk, cheese, ice cream, and butter. Some vegetable oils are high in saturated fats such as coconut, palm kernel, and palm oil. Saturated fat also includes trans fat, which is found in shortening, margarine, baked and fried foods, doughnuts, and other processed foods made with or fried in partially hydrogenated oil. Trans fats are also found naturally in some animal products, like dairy products.

Most of the fat that you eat should be *polyunsaturated* (PUFA) or *monounsaturated fat* (MUFA), and oils are the major source for both. These fats do not raise LDL (bad) blood cholesterol levels. In addition to containing essential fatty acids, PUFA and MUFA are the major sources of vitamin E in a typical diet. Nuts, fish, cooking oil, and salad dressings provide enough oil to achieve the recommended daily allowance for these nutrients. As previously stated, consuming fat or oil is needed for health. However, be aware that one tablespoon of fat or oil contains approximately 120 calories, an amount that should be limited to balance total calorie intake.

Water

Water and fluids are essential for good health and necessary for life. Every body cell needs water to function. Water helps regulate temperature, move nutrients through the body, and remove waste. Cancer treatments like chemotherapy and radiation can leave you dehydrated, and some drugs can even damage the kidneys if they are not flushed out of the system. If you lose fluids through vomiting or diarrhea, important nutrients and minerals are lost, and normal body functioning can become dangerously out of balance. You do get some water from the foods that you eat, but it is also a good idea to drink around six to eight glasses of water a day. Along with drinking more water, patients can try sports drinks, like Gatorade, that can also help to maintain electrolyte balance.

If you find it hard to drink enough water (chemotherapy can make even water taste strange), consider increasing fluid intake through soups. Adding a bit of flavor from chicken soup, for example, may make it easier for you to achieve proper hydration.

Vitamins and Minerals

Vitamins such as A, C, D, and E are important nutrients that are needed in small amounts by the body. They promote cell metabolism and help the body to grow and stay strong. Vitamins aid in good vision, healthy skin, nails, and hair. The following list of vitamins function as *antioxidants* in the body. Antioxidants protect cells from the damaging effects of *free radicals*. Free radicals cause damage to cells and might contribute to the development of cardiovascular disease and cancer.

- *Vitamin C* is found in many fruits and vegetables, especially oranges, grapefruits, and peppers. Vitamin C is an antioxidant that binds to free radicals in the body, preventing them from attaching to normal cells. Vitamin C is recommended to prevent cardiovascular problems like heart attack and stroke, osteoarthritis, and cataracts or macular degeneration. Select studies have found that women who consume high amounts of vitamin C have a lower risk of breast cancer; however, research in general has not shown a strong connection. A recent review of thirty-eight studies on vitamin C and cancer in general concluded that vitamin C cannot prevent or treat cancer. Very high doses of vitamin C can interfere with blood thinners, and there is some concern that high doses may reduce the effectiveness of certain cancer treatments such as chemotherapy and radiation.

- *Beta-carotene* is a powerful antioxidant that is found in carrots and green leafy vegetables such as beet greens, spinach, and broccoli. Because eating fruits and vegetables has been associated with a reduced risk of cancer, it was thought that taking a supplement of high-dose beta-carotene might protect against cancer. Unfortunately, results of three major clinical trials show that this is not the case. In two studies, high-dose supplements of beta-carotene given to prevent lung cancer were found to instead increase the lung cancer risk in cigarette smokers. The third study found no harm or benefit from the supplement. From this we should consider that eating fruits and vegetables containing beta-carotene might be helpful, but high-dose supplements of beta-carotene supplements should be avoided.

- *Vitamin D* is a fat-soluble vitamin that is found naturally in very few foods. It is involved in a number of processes essential to good health, including: improved muscle strength and immune function, reduced inflammation, increased calcium absorption, and protection from osteoporosis. Vitamin D is obtained through skin exposure to ultraviolet radiation and through diet, particularly fortified products such as milk, cereals, and supplements. Many Americans do not get enough vitamin D. There is growing evidence that vitamin D may have helpful effects on some types of cancer, including colon, prostate, and breast cancers. For many years, studies have shown that people who are less exposed to sunlight and have lower levels of vitamin D as a result are more likely to develop breast cancer and other forms of cancer. More recently, some research has found that calcium and vitamin D may help protect premenopausal women against breast cancer, but more studies are needed.

- *Vitamin E* is a fat-soluble antioxidant found naturally in some foods, added to others, and available as a dietary supplement. It is involved in immune function. A number of research trials that attempted to associate vitamin E intake with cancer incidence have generally been inconclusive. In one study, male smokers who took vitamin E had a lower risk of prostate cancer, but additional studies have not found the same link. While studies are ongoing, it appears for now that there is no benefit from vitamin E in reducing cancer risk.

Minerals are chemicals that help regulate body processes. For example, potassium helps with nerve and muscle function, and iron carries oxygen to all of your cells.

Calcium is important for strong teeth and bones. Calcium supplements can strengthen bones and prevent osteoporosis. Bone loss is of special concern to breast cancer patients who are taking aromatase inhibitors, since bone loss is one side effect of AIs. Calcium can also help to prevent the weakening of bones that can occur with certain chemotherapy medications. It is helpful in controlling blood pressure, and several studies suggest that calcium may help reduce the risk of breast and colorectal cancer. Additional research found that vitamin D combined with calcium may help protect premenopausal women from developing breast cancer, but more research is needed.

Dairy products are excellent sources of calcium, as are leafy green vegetables such as kale, collards, beet greens, cabbage, brussels sprouts, and broccoli. Additional sources of calcium include tofu, molasses, and almonds. Most kinds of beans, fish (such as salmon with bones and halibut), berries, raisins, and some grains are also good sources you can include in your diet. Calcium supplements are available in a number of different forms. Some are more absorbable than others, including calcium citrate, or microcrystalline hydroxyapatite concentrate (MCHC), which is a crystalline complex providing calcium, phosphorus, and organic factors naturally present in healthy bones. Some calcium preparations have a small amount of vitamin D added.

If you eat a balanced diet with enough calories and protein, you will most likely get the right amount of vitamins and minerals. But eating a balanced diet can be hard to do when you are being treated for breast cancer, and some treatments may compromise your body's supplies of vitamins and minerals. To ensure you are getting all the essential vitamins and minerals that you need, you may consider including a multivitamin/mineral supplement. Avoid high-dose multivitamins as there is concern that high-dose antioxidants could interfere with your breast cancer treatment. One regular multivitamin per day is the best choice to meet your nutrient needs, and remember to check with your doctor before making changes or additions to your current diet.

Herbs and Other Supplements

Breast cancer treatments such as chemotherapy or hormonal therapy can cause women to experience menopausal symptoms such as hot flashes. Many patients turn to alternative therapies such as herbs or other supplements to try and reduce these symptoms. It's important to do some investigating before adding any supplement to your diet, particularly if you are currently undergoing breast cancer treatment. Some supplements may change the way medications or radiation work in your body and may even make the treatments less effective. Before deciding on any dietary supplement be sure to talk to your physician or registered dietitian so that you fully understand the risks and benefits. A number of alternative remedies commonly used by breast cancer patients are described below.

Black cohosh has many other names: baneberry, bugwort, black snakeroot, cimicfuga, rattle root, squaw root, RemiSure, and Remifemin. It may be effective to relieve menopausal symptoms, particularly hot flashes. In one clinical study black cohosh provided no more relief from hot flashes than a placebo (sugar pill). Researchers suggest that black cohosh may act on estrogen receptors in some way and could possibly be associated with reduced risk of breast cancer. Until more is known, women at high risk for breast cancer or those who have already been diagnosed should consult their oncologist prior to using black cohosh. It appears that black cohosh is safe at the recommended doses, but possible side effects include autoimmune hepatitis and liver damage. The usual dose is 1 milligram twice a day.

Dong quai also goes by the names *Angelica sinensis*, Chinese angelica, dang gui, danggui, dong qua, ligustilides, and tan kuei. Dong quai may lessen menopausal symptoms, high blood pressure, anemia, constipation, and allergic reactions. There has not been enough research done to determine if dong quai is safe or effective for relieving menopausal symtoms and no studies have included breast cancer patients. Using dong quai for a short time is considered safe, but long-term use has not been studied. The usual dose is 4.5 grams/day.

Flaxseed or flaxseed oil is also known as *Linum usitatissimum* or linseed. Flaxseed is a grain found in some multi-grain bread, cereal, or breakfast bars. It contains compounds that may have a weak estrogen effect. This weak estrogen compound may bind to a breast cell's estrogen receptor blocking the body's stronger estrogen from binding. In this way, flaxseed compounds might work against breast cancers that depend on estrogen for growth. Research into the association between flaxseed and breast cancer is small and has focused on animal studies. Additional research in humans is needed to examine this connection further. Flaxseed is high in fiber and its oil is a good source of omega-3 fatty acids. Flaxseed can help with your cholesterol, and can also reduce constipation. Dietitians recommend eating 1–2 tablespoons of ground flaxseed per day, and be sure to drink plenty of water.

Green tea is also known as *Camellia sinensis*, green tea polyphenols, or ECGC (epigallocatechin 3-gallate). The natural polyphenols found in green tea leaves serve as natural antioxidants and may prevent cell damage that could lead to cancer. In laboratory and animal studies EGCG, the primary polyphenol in green tea, has been shown to limit growth of breast cancer cells. A study of Asian-American women found that those who drank more green tea were less likely to develop breast cancer, although much more research is needed regarding the connection between green tea and breast cancer.

Green tea has less caffeine than black tea or coffee—about 25 milligrams per cup, but if you are sensitive to caffeine it might make you jittery or nauseated. The usual dose is 3–4 cups per day. One cup of tea contains 80–100 milligrams of polyphenol depending on the size of the cup and the strength of the brewed tea.

Red clover is also known as daidzein, genistein, isoflavone, phytoestrogen, purple clover, trefoil, trifolium beebread, or clovone. This herb is used to treat menopausal symptoms such as hot flashes. The active ingredient in red clover is phytoestrogen. According to research, red clover may interfere with hormonal therapy drugs and is not recommended for women with ER-positive breast cancer. Reports indicate red clover is not effective in treating hot flashes although some women do report mild improvement. Side effects include rashes, headache, and nausea and its use may increase bleeding, especially if combined with anti-clotting medications. There is no standard dose; however, an extract of 40 to 160 milligrams has been used to treat hot flashes.

The Relationship between Soy and Breast Cancer

✎ Plants produce compounds called *phytochemicals* (plant chemicals). Phytochemicals found in fruits, vegetables, grains, and beans are believed to protect cells from damage that could lead to cancer. By increasing your daily intake of plant-based foods, some researchers believe you can reduce your cancer risk, although more research is needed to find out which phytochemicals are most beneficial and in what combination. While researchers have identified more than 4,000 phytochemicals, only about 150 have been well studied. Some of the better known phytochemicals include flavonoids, antioxidants, carotenoids, anthocyanins, sulfides, phytosterols, and isoflavones.

The soy plant produces isoflavones, which are weak *phytoestrogens*. One of these phytoestrogens, genistein, is about 1/100,000 as strong as your body's estrogen, and it has the ability to bind to estrogen receptors in the breast. There are many more phytochemicals in soy, including protein kinase inhibitors (which help maintain normal cell growth), phenolic acid and phytates (which act as antioxidants), and phytosterols and saponins (which help regulate cholesterol).

For people who do not eat meat, soy is promoted as a healthy protein alternative. Much of the research into the effects of soy on cancer risk reduction has come from observing population groups such as the Japanese, who begin eating soy at an early age and eat large quantities of it—about ten times as much as the typical woman in the United States. Results from studies examining the relationship between soy and breast cancer have been mixed.

The possible connection between soy and breast cancer is complicated by several factors. Women in Asia consume soy as their main protein source and only small amounts of beef, chicken, and pork. This means they get far less animal fat in their diets, among other possibly unhealthy things. The Asian woman's lifestyle includes even more differences: more fresh vegetables are consumed, most are close to their ideal body weight, they are less likely to drink significant amounts of alcohol, and they tend to be more physically active. These factors combined produce a healthier lifestyle and a lower risk of breast cancer in Asian women.

Soy isoflavones may have an effect on hormone receptor–positive breast cancers because they may interfere with hormonal therapy's ability to function properly. Until further evidence is found, many doctors recommend that women who take hormonal therapy or who have estrogen receptor–positive breast cancer do not take high-concentration soy supplements.

It has been suggested that soy isoflavones may relieve menopausal symptoms, including hot flashes, by mimicking the action of estrogen. In some studies, postmenopausal women who ate high amounts of soy (20 to 60 g per day) had fewer and less intense hot flashes and night sweats than those with low soy intakes. Other research studies have not found this to be the case.

In general, moderate amounts of soy foods can be included as part of a balanced diet. Soy comes in many forms, including tofu, beans (also known as edamame), soy milk, miso, and soy powder. One to three half-cup servings of soy a day is similar to an average Japanese woman's daily soy intake. If you are taking hormonal therapy, ask your doctor about how much soy you can eat.

In summary, we believe that the nutrients that you give to your cells are an extremely important adjunct to your treatment and recovery. Adequate fluid replacement is critically important in flushing toxins that result from cancer treatment and cell death out of your system. Often, when you don't feel up to replenishing your nutrients and fluids, that's the very time when you most need to do so. We recommend a nutritional plan as part of your cancer treatment, and you may want to consult a registered dietitian. Information to help you locate a dietitian in your area is provided in the Resources section.

15

·······

❧

Life after Breast Cancer Diagnosis

BECOMING A SURVIVOR

If you are just beginning your journey with breast cancer, you may want to put this chapter aside for a while and come back at a later time once you get through your *acute treatment phase*—and you will! For most women, breast cancer is a life-altering experience. Statistically, you are joining three million U.S. women who are also survivors and with whom you share many experiences relating to this disease. This chapter addresses issues of survivorship: fear of recurrence and health screening; health maintenance such as bone health; hormonal concerns and sexuality; financial and insurance issues; spirituality and stewardship.

Fear of Recurrence and Health Monitoring

❧ A majority of women are cured of their breast cancer—more than 80 percent! To me, *cured* means that you live the rest of your life without recurrence, and you die of something other than breast cancer, it is hoped in the distant future and beyond your eightieth year. But we do not know with *absolute confidence* if you are cured. My hope is that by using this manual and with the help of your medical team you have received optimal treatment and you have given yourself the best possible chance. All survivors have some anxiety about recurrence. Early on, the everyday aches and maladies of living can rekindle this anxiety. Risk of recurrence does decrease over time; however, there is no absolute length of time that guarantees cure. One certainly celebrates five- and ten-year anniversaries. We know that women with triple-negative and Her2 types of breast cancer are usually safe after three years and that women with Luminal A or Luminal B cancers can relapse after five years but rarely after ten. I should point out that women who do relapse with metastatic disease often have long-term survival with current and evolving treatment strategies. The management and prognosis of metastatic breast cancer can be very similar to other chronic diseases of aging, such as diabetes, chronic lung disease, and heart disease.

A major controversy among the medical establishment is how closely survivors should be monitored for systemic recurrence. There is no question that survivors need annual breast screening to monitor for local recurrence or a second breast cancer. Women receiving adjuvant hormonal treatment such as tamoxifen or aromatase inhibitors are usually followed by their oncologist every three to six months with examinations and blood tests until the treatment is complete. We do not believe in routine radiologic scanning (CT, PET, and bone scans) unless there is a persistent symptom or an abnormal blood test. We think that women with a history of breast cancer who have remaining breast tissue have a modest increased risk of a second breast cancer and require annual diagnostic mammograms. For women with increased breast density, we also recommend an annual breast MRI.

Bone Health

Bone health is a major issue for breast cancer survivors. It is important to be proactive in helping women to protect their bone mass and guard against osteoporosis in later life. Breast cancer survivors have treatment issues that make them vulnerable to accelerated bone loss, including: (1) chemotherapy and chemotherapy-induced menopause, (2) estrogen deficiency and the lack of hormone replacement therapy, (3) aromatase inhibitor (AI) treatment, and (4) vitamin D deficiency, which has been associated with breast cancer. It is important to monitor bone health in order to intervene appropriately. We recommend that our patients have a baseline vitamin D serum level and a bone density exam. We also advise taking supplemental vitamin D and calcium supplementation (see chapter 14), with lifestyle modifications, including smoking cessation and weight-bearing exercise.

Several drugs are beneficial for the treatment of osteoporosis, including the bisphosphanates (Fosamax, Boniva, Zometa) and a recent FDA-approved drug, Denosumab. These drugs do have side effects. The bisphosphanates contribute to *gastroesophageal reflux disease* (*GERD*) and can rarely cause unusual fractures in the middle of the *femur* (thigh bone). Both classes of drugs can also lead to *osteonecrosis* of the jaw (*ONJ*), although this too is rare.

ONJ, when it occurs, usually follows a dental procedure such as a tooth extraction or root canal. With *osteopenia* (significant bone density decrease but with no risk of fracture), we recommend conservative management with vitamin D and calcium supplementation and exercise. However, if a woman is on an AI, or if she continues to lose bone mass on the conservative treatment, we will add a bisphosphanate or Denosumab after a thorough baseline dental exam.

Gynecologic Health, Sexuality, and Hormone Replacement Therapy (HRT)

There are often major concerns for the breast cancer patient around gynecologic issues, particularly for younger *premenopausal* or *perimenopausal* patients with Luminal A or Luminal B (hormone receptor–positive) cancer who are receiving adjuvant hormonal therapy. It is estimated that as high as 50 percent of these patients will discontinue hormonal therapy (increasing their risk of recurrence) because of side effects, many of which are related to estrogen deficiency and menopausal symptoms. The medical community needs to help women suffering from these unpleasant side effects before they *throw in the towel* on this very important and potentially lifesaving treatment. The AIs were first marketed by the pharmaceutical industry as superior to tamoxifen, and while the two classes of hormonal therapy are fairly equal in efficacy, their side effects are different. Although it is true that the AIs don't increase the risk of *uterine hyperplasia* (a rare but serious side effect that can lead to uterine cancer) or increase the risk of *venous thrombosis* (a blood clot in a vein)—both of which are attributed to tamoxifen—the complete estrogen blockade caused by the AIs can lead to side effects that are intolerable for some women. Common complaints are *arthralgias* (joint and muscle aches), loss of sexual desire, vaginal thinning, and vasomotor symptoms (hot flashes). For some postmenopausal women, tamoxifen in combination with vaginal estrogen can be a much better tolerated regimen in spite of the rare serious side effects that we can monitor for.

HRT in breast cancer survivors is a controversial and complex subject. In 2001 the Women's Health Initiative (WHI) Study reported an increased risk of breast cancer in women taking a combination of estrogen and progesterone. The same study reported that women who'd had a hysterectomy and were taking estrogen alone had no increase in breast cancer, had increased bone density, had decreased incidence of colon cancer, and received no benefit in cardiovascular or Alzheimer prevention. Follow-up reports in 2009 further confirmed these findings.

The use of HRT in breast cancer survivors has been discouraged, especially in women who survived hormone receptor–positive cancer. This is in spite of the fact that a vast majority, more than 80 percent, of these patients are cured. Added to this is my belief that if a woman has a systemic relapse after initiating HRT, the HRT has not caused the relapse. The cancer was there and may have recurred somewhat earlier because of the estrogen stimulation. As stated in chapter 8, we need a safe, SERM-like hormone replacement that is safe for breasts and good for bones, et cetera.

In the meantime the medical community should provide individualized, supportive therapy around quality-of-life issues for women who are undergoing adjuvant hormonal therapy or who are beyond active treatment. For some women, homeopathic remedies, herbs, and SSRIs are ineffective in controlling symptoms. For women who are so symptomatic that they are willing to abandon adjuvant tamoxifen therapy in spite of the survival benefit, I will sometimes add low-dose estrogen with excellent relief of symptoms. There is no clinical trial to support this approach, but I think it is worthy of closer evaluation. Theoretically, it should be safe (excluding uterine stimulation) because we know tamoxifen is effective in preventing systemic relapse in premenopausal women who are producing their own estrogen.

Fertility

For young women with breast cancer, fertility can be an important issue. As modern women delay childbearing, breast cancer can suddenly jeopardize a woman's or a couple's ability to have children. A large percentage of young women have hormone-negative cancer (triple-negative or Her2-positive) requiring chemotherapy, but not requiring long-term hormonal therapy that would cause an extended delay of pregnancy. Chemotherapy can affect endocrine function (hormone production) of the ovary in premenopausal women receiving this therapy. The degree of the dysfunction depends on the intensity and type of chemotherapy and the health and age of the woman's ovaries. Most women under age thirty-five will have transient interruption of ovulation due to the chemotherapy exposure. Usually within six months and rarely up to one year after completing chemotherapy, ovulation and menstrual cycling resume.

Women entering their forties have fewer remaining eggs and older ovaries, and their fertility may be more affected by chemotherapy: there is a small but real chance of permanent cessation of ovulation and menstrual periods (premature menopause). Egg harvesting with embryo storage is an option. Our policy is to offer premenopausal women interested in fertility the opportunity to see a gynecologist who specializes in fertility medicine. If patients elect to undergo this treatment, there will be some delay in beginning the breast cancer treatment, so it is important for physicians to make this referral as early as possible.

Stress and Breast Cancer

✖ Many of my patients ask me this question: "Dr. Link, did stress cause or contribute to my breast cancer?" And the follow-up question: "If the answer is yes, where does that leave me, now that I am even more stressed because of the cancer diagnosis!" In spite of considerable literature from the 1980s linking stressful events to a diagnosis of cancer, I do not believe that stress in any way causes breast cancer. The old literature does not stand up to scientific scrutiny. While some animal studies have found a relationship between chronic stress exposure and decreased immune function, I do not believe that decreased immunity has a major role in the development of breast cancer. We do not know why women get breast cancer and why the incidence has increased substantially over the last thirty years, except in two instances. We know from epidemiologists that long-term exposure (greater than five years) to an estrogen/progesterone combination increases a woman's risk of Luminal B breast cancer. This is approximately a 20 percent increase over a similar population of women not taking the hormones. We also know that women who have inherited either a BRCA1 or a BRCA2 gene mutation from their parents have about a 50 percent risk of developing breast cancer. But that's it.

Life is stressful. Getting breast cancer is stressful. I believe continuous unrelieved stress is bad, and people who feel hopeless are more prone to illness—stomach ulcers, high blood pressure, and various addictions. Your breast cancer, although stressful, is not hopeless, and you should have a plan that will allow you to survive. Some women with a new breast cancer diagnosis are able to look at their stressful life situations and make significant changes—switch to a less stressful a job or career, end a difficult relationship, or restructure a financial burden, for example. These are usually good things to do and free up energy to address the important task at hand. While I don't want to discourage anyone from making important and healthy changes, it is important to remember that stress did not cause your cancer. A diagnosis of cancer can be a great motivator and a change agent, but I do not believe that women have caused their breast cancer by being overstressed, and we certainly encourage women to seek supportive networks or professional help when needed.

Obesity and Breast Cancer

✗ Obesity is a major problem for our modern society, and it is associated with increasing a woman's risk of cardiovascular disease, diabetes, and breast cancer. Obesity and cigarette smoking are two of the most important risk factors for premature death in the United States today.

To accurately measure body weight, we prefer to use *body mass index* (*BMI*). BMI is a measure of body fat that is based on a person's height and weight. There are a number of different Web sites that can help you calculate BMI; for example, the National Heart, Lung, and Blood Institute BMI Calculator can be found at http://www.nhlbisupport .com/bmi. A BMI of 18 or less is considered underweight; 18.5 to 24.9 is normal; 25 to 29.9 is overweight; 30 and over is obese. Sixty percent of Americans are overweight or obese. Breast cancer recurrence risk increases with a BMI over 25; a number of possible reasons for this correlation have been proposed. Increased body fat results in: (1) higher estrogen levels, (2) elevated insulin levels due to insulin resistance, (3) elevated levels of insulin-like growth factor and other *cytokines* (indicators of immune response).

It is not easy to lose weight. Ninety-five percent of individuals with

BMI greater than 35 (morbidly obese) will fail to lose a substantial amount of weight. For these people, the risk of premature death is high enough that gastric bypass is a major consideration. The medical community has begun to have a more realistic expectation around calorie restriction and exercise in patients with chronic obesity. In fact, Medicare recently lowered the requirement for lap band surgery to a BMI of 30.

Often a breast cancer diagnosis provides motivation for women to try and lose weight, but it is still not easy. Women requiring chemotherapy often gain rather than lose, and the same is true with adjuvant hormonal therapy. While you are undergoing your cancer treatments, it is important to eat a healthy, balanced diet in order to provide the nutrients you need to maintain energy and help your body heal. It is best to begin a weight loss program after treatments are completed.

Studies provide evidence that physical exercise decreases the incidence of breast cancer. The goal is to achieve weight reduction through diet (caloric restriction) and exercise. This is difficult to do alone without significant changes in lifestyle. I believe the best approach to achieve lifestyle changes is to seek professional nutrition counseling from a registered dietitian or other nutrition health professional, enroll in an organized weight-loss program, and be sure to include exercise as a part of your healthy lifestyle routine.

Alcohol

A fair number of epidemiologic studies have explored the link between alcohol and breast cancer. There is strong evidence to suggest that there may be a connection between alcohol consumption, breast cancer incidence, and the risk of recurrence. If you search the Internet for *breast cancer and alcohol*, you will find over one million references. The data, however, are conflicting and difficult to interpret and for the most part rely on *retrospective studies*. If you choose to drink alcohol, it should be consumed in moderation (no more than three to five six-ounce glasses of beer or wine per week). In my opinion the Life After Cancer Epidemiology (LACE) Study, conducted at the Kaiser Permanente HMO System in Northern California, is one of the best to date. The study results seem to indicate that there was an increased risk of breast cancer recurrence in women who drank more than six ounces of alcohol per day. However, when results were more closely examined, it was only *postmenopausal obese women* who were at increased risk. Premenopausal and postmenopausal women with BMI less than 25 had no increase in risk. I interpret this to mean that moderate alcohol consumption is *not a major risk factor* for breast cancer, and it may not be a risk factor at all. The culprit may well be obesity, as we previously discussed.

Financial Concerns and Health Insurance

✀ Earlier in this chapter we discussed stress in relation to breast cancer. I cannot imagine anything more stressful than receiving a diagnosis of breast cancer and not being confident that one has reliable access to care and treatment. In the wealthiest nation in the world this should not be an issue, but it is. For the increasing percentage of women without health insurance, gaining access to breast cancer treatment is a daunting task. Many states have programs for uninsured women with newly diagnosed breast cancer, and I recommend that these women go to a local facility that can direct them to treatment. There are resources available—comprehensive cancer centers, university teaching hospitals, and local community hospitals that have both teaching and research programs involved in the diagnosis and treatment of breast cancer. These institutions also have social workers or other health advocates available in addition to programs for women without financial resources. The Resources section of this book provides Web sites and contact information that can help in this regard.

Many women are eligible for research protocols that are supported by the government (National Cancer Institute) and the pharmaceutical industry. There are large and small foundations that help women in need. Most of the pharmaceutical companies have assistance programs to help women who are uninsured or underinsured.

Even for women with health insurance, there are financial concerns and issues. "Will I be able to work and support myself during treatment" is a common worry. "Will my insurance cover the treatment I need?" Once you connect to a treatment center, these issues can be addressed with the help of the staff.

No woman in this country should go without proper treatment. The resources are available; the challenge is finding the connections.

Maintaining and Updating Your Medical Records

In this manual we recommend that you become educated and actively participate in your breast cancer care. To help achieve this goal we encourage you to maintain a copy of your medical records from initial diagnosis through treatment to follow-up care. This can be simply accomplished by gathering paper copies of your documents into a large three-ring notebook that has been divided into tabbed sections. Alternatively, you can subscribe to a Web-based electronic application that allows you to enter and access your health records by computer at any time. It makes sense to begin collecting your medical records right from the start, rather than trying to do so later when it becomes more difficult to retrieve records, reports, and images. We believe this is critically important in an evolving medical system. To help you in this process, we have created a *breast cancer specific* electronic application that can be found on our Web site at: www.drjohn linkbreastcancercare.com. Whether you use this electronic format or you create your own, keeping track of your breast cancer medical history will help you to stay informed and allow you to be more connected to your breast cancer journey.

Advocacy and Stewardship

One of the brightest and most heartening things I have observed in my career as a breast oncologist has been the connecting, supporting, and philanthropy that occurs among women with breast cancer. This benevolent movement has generated major organizations and numerous support groups. The *sisterhood* with its pink ribbon logo is everywhere. Surely you will receive some benefit from this movement; perhaps from joining a support group, becoming a volunteer at your treatment center, or enrolling in research funded by a "breast cancer walk" or "run." In my experience women deal with this illness in different ways. The current task at hand is for you to get optimal treatment that will give you the best chance for a cure. Once you complete the "acute" treatment phase and become a *survivor*, you may want to become involved in some way in the breast cancer movement. My advice to patients is to *feel no pressure* to get involved; you should do so only when or if you are ready. Remember, there will be plenty of opportunities to join or volunteer. You are going to be a survivor for the rest of your life.

16
. . . . . .
❧

Conclusion

In this manual we have attempted to give you a foundation to launch you on your journey to a breast cancer cure. We have presented a large amount of new information that has become available since the previous edition was published. The new classification of breast cancer, based on genomic differences in cancer cells, is particularly relevant because it leads to markedly different treatment decisions. Our understanding of breast cancer is expanding extremely rapidly. The information in this book will be current for a very short period as we continue to unravel the cancer cell's DNA. New, "targeted" agents will be developed based on this new research and will be added to the half-dozen targeted drugs currently in use or being tested in early-stage breast cancer. At the time of the previous edition, there was only one targeted drug, Herceptin. We hope new research will ultimately lead to the discovery of the causes of breast cancer, causes that have been so elusive to researchers until now.

We discussed the importance of becoming involved in understanding your choices and the benefits of getting a second opinion. Second opinions become even more important as new techniques and treatments move rapidly from *research* into clinical practice.

Breast cancer is scary. Much of this fear stems from our inability to predict absolute outcomes in spite of our analysis with computers and genomic tests. Decisions may involve taking *risks* that must be weighed against *benefit*. Perhaps our most important task is to help you understand the risks and benefits of decisions that we are asking you to make.

It may be hard for you to believe, but you will get through this. In spite of the fear and uncertainty, the pain and discomfort, a diagnosis of breast cancer can have a "silver lining." Like other existential crises, it has the ability to help one refocus on what is important, what is sacred, and what is joyful. Breast cancer will force you to make decisions involving risk (there is no escape by default). You have the opportunity *to be afraid*, to be heroic, to take risks, and most important, *to survive*.

Anna Quindlen in her wonderful little book, *A Short Guide to a Happy Life*, describes her journey of transformation after her mother's death.

> I learned to love the journey, not the destination. I learned that this is not a dress rehearsal, and that today is the only guarantee you get.
>
> I learned to look at all the good in the world and to try to give some back, because I believed in it completely and utterly. And I tried to do that, in part, by telling others what I had learned . . . By telling them this: Consider the lilies of the field. Look at the fuzz on a baby's ear. Read in the backyard with the sun on your face. Learn to be happy. And think of life as a terminal illness, because if you do, you will live it with joy and passion as it ought to be lived.

We hope that this survival manual will aid you on this "unchosen journey" of breast cancer and will help you to live long, be happy, and survive well.

Resources

The Internet can be a great source of information about breast health and breast cancer. Every day more and more information becomes available and in a very few minutes you can learn about the latest in breast cancer screening or research, locate a clinical research trial, or confirm that a surgeon is board certified.

But how can you be sure that the information on a Web site is accurate and safe? Obtaining a referral from a trusted source is a good way to ensure that you are getting up-to-date information. You can also rely on well-known and trusted sites such as the National Cancer Institute (www.cancer.gov), the American Cancer Society (www.cancer.org), and even large university Web sites.

To help you get started we have included a number of trusted Web sites below that we believe can provide you with a wealth of information, education, and support.

Nonprofit Health Organizations

American Cancer Society (ACS)
www.cancer.org
The American Cancer Society is a nationwide, community-based, voluntary health organization dedicated to eliminating cancer as a major health problem by preventing cancer, saving lives, and diminishing suffering from cancer, through research, education, advocacy, and service. E-mail or call their helpline for cancer-related questions and for links to other resources.

BreastCancer.org
www.breastcancer.org
Breastcancer.org is a nonprofit organization dedicated to providing the most reliable, complete, and up-to-date information about breast cancer. Its mission is to help women and families make sense of complex medical and personal information about breast cancer, so they can make the best decisions for their lives. On this site you will find reliable health information available for those affected by breast cancer and concerned about breast health.

Breast Cancer Care and Research Fund
www.breastcancercare.org
The Breast Cancer Care and Research Fund is a nonprofit organization that provides information and education to make breast cancer patients, their supporters, and the lay public more knowledgeable about breast cancer, treatments, and research.

Cancer Care, Inc.
www.cancercare.org
CancerCare, Inc. helps individuals and families cope with and manage the emotional and practical challenges resulting from cancer. Services for patients, survivors, loved ones, caregivers, and the bereaved include counseling and support groups, educational publications and workshops, and financial assistance. Professional oncology social workers provide assistance free of charge.

Cancer Support Community
www.cancersupportcommunity.org
The mission of the Cancer Support Community (CSC) is to ensure that all people impacted by cancer are empowered by knowledge, strengthened by action, and sustained by community. The CSC is an international nonprofit dedicated to providing support, education, and hope to people affected by cancer. This large global network of psychosocial oncology mental health professionals brings the highest quality cancer support to the millions of people touched by cancer. Support services are available through professionally led community-based centers, hospitals, community oncology practices, and online, so that no one has to face cancer alone.

Kids Konnected
www.kidskonnected.org
This nonprofit provides education, understanding, and support for children who have a parent with cancer or who have lost a parent to cancer. The Kids

Konnected Web site includes a 24-hour hotline, youth leadership, camps, and social events.

Living Beyond Breast Cancer
www.lbbc.org

Living Beyond Breast Cancer (LBBC) is a national education and support organization, whose goal is to improve the quality of life for breast cancer patients and to encourage patients to take an active role in ongoing recovery or management of the disease, regardless of educational background, social support, or financial means. LBCC offers programs and services to women affected by breast cancer, caregivers, and health care providers. They offer specialized programs and services for the newly diagnosed, young women, women with advanced breast cancer, women at high risk for developing the disease, and African American and Latina women. Programs are available for caregivers and health care professionals to help better meet the needs of women affected by breast cancer.

National Breast Cancer Coalition
www.stopbreastcancer2020.org

The mission of the National Breast Cancer Coalition (NBCC) is to eradicate breast cancer. The NBCC encourages all those concerned about the disease to become advocates for action and change. The coalition informs, trains, and directs patients and others in effective advocacy efforts. Nationwide, women and men are increasing the awareness of breast cancer public policy by participating in legislative, scientific, and regulatory decisions, promoting positive media coverage, and actively working to raise public awareness. In 2010 NBCC launched a bold initiative, *Breast Cancer Deadline 2020*, a call to action for policy-makers, researchers, breast cancer advocates, and other stakeholders to end the disease by 2020.

National Lymphedema Network
www.lymphnet.org

This international nonprofit group provides referrals, education, and guidance to lymphedema patients, health care professionals, and the general public. The National Lymphedema Network publishes a quarterly newsletter and holds a biennial conference for health care professionals.

National Patient Advocate Foundation
www.npaf.org

The National Patient Advocate Foundation (NPAF) is a national nonprofit organization providing the patient voice in improving access to, and reimbursement for, high-quality health care through regulatory and legislative reform at the state and federal levels. NPAF translates the experience of millions of patients who have been helped by our companion, Patient Advocate Foundation, which provides professional case management services to individuals facing barriers to health care access for chronic and disabling diseases, medical debt crisis, and employment-related issues at no cost.

SHARE
www.sharecancersupport.org

The mission of SHARE is to create and sustain a supportive network and community of women affected by breast or ovarian cancer. SHARE brings women, their families, and friends together with others who have experienced breast or ovarian cancer, and provides participants with the opportunity to receive and exchange information, support, strength, and hope. SHARE's work focuses on empowerment, education, and advocacy, to bring about better health care, an improved quality of life, and a cure for these diseases.

Susan G. Komen for the Cure
www.komen.org

Susan G. Komen for the Cure is the world's largest grassroots network of breast cancer survivors and activists that is fighting to save lives, empower people, ensure quality care for all, and energize science to find the cure. Its Web site provides education to help understand breast cancer as well as information about research and research trials, numerous way to get involved, and links to many other valuable breast cancer resources.

Y-Me National Breast Cancer Organization
www.y-me.org

Y-Me is a national nonprofit founded in 1978 with the mission to ensure, through information, empowerment, and peer support, that no one faces breast cancer alone. Peer support is the cornerstone of the Y-Me Breast Cancer Organization and peer counselors are available around the clock, 365 days a year.

Young Survival Coalition
www.youngsurvival.org

The Young Survival Coalition (YSC) is an international organization dedicated to the critical issues unique to young women diagnosed with breast cancer. YSC offers resources, connections, and outreach so women feel supported, empowered, and hopeful.

Professional Resources

American College of Radiology
www.acr.org

The American College of Radiology Web site includes information for and about radiologists, radiation oncologists, medical physicists, interventional radiologists, and nuclear medicine physicians. Patients have a say in who provides their health care and where to receive it. A core element of the ACR's mission is to maximize the quality and safety of patient care by providing resources to help one make informed decisions. The ACR devotes its resources to making imaging safe, effective, and accessible to those who need it. This Web site provides valuable patient information regarding radiation, imaging, and patient safety issues.

American Society of Plastic and Reconstructive Surgeons (ASPS)
www.plasticsurgery.org

The American Society of Plastic and Reconstructive Surgeons publishes numerous informational brochures and maintains this Web site to provide public education about plastic surgery. This site includes news on the latest advances and techniques in plastic and reconstructive surgeries and details of specific surgical procedures, including how to prepare for surgery, the types of anesthesia used, and how long recovery takes. Look for answers to the most frequently asked questions about plastic surgery and statistics.

American Dietetic Association
www.eatright.org

The American Dietetic Association (ADA) is the world's largest organization of food and nutrition professionals. ADA is committed to improving the nation's health and advancing the profession of dietetics through research, education, and advocacy. On the ADA Web site you will find the latest food and nutrition information, hot topics in nutrition, nutritional guidance for different stages of life, and disease management and prevention, as well as food safety and links to many other resources. The ADA Web site can also assist in locating a registered dietitian where you live.

Breastlink Medical Group
www.breastlink.com

Breastlink Medical Group is dedicated to deliver optimal care for women with breast cancer. The Optimal Care program is delivered through a team-based approach that includes radiologists, oncologists, surgeons, and pathologists focused specifically on the diagnosis, care, and treatment of breast cancer. Breastlink offers a comprehensive second-opinion service based on the team approach. To request a second opinion, please visit our Web site above. There you will find complete instructions on how to obtain a timely comprehensive opinion from our Optimal Care Breast Center.

National Society of Genetic Counselors
www.nsgc.org

The National Society of Genetic Counselors is an association of professionals who help people understand and adapt to the medical, psychological, and familial implications of genetic contributions to disease. This process includes: (1) Interpretation of family and medical histories to assess the chance of disease occurrence or recurrence, (2) Education about inheritance, testing, management, prevention, resources, and research, and (3) Counseling to promote informed choices and adaptation to the risk or condition. In addition to providing education, this Web site can assist in locating a genetic counselor in your area. (For an additional resource please see *My Family Health Portrait* under Government Agencies below.)

Government Agencies

Clinical Trials
www.clinicaltrials.org

The National Institutes of Health (NIH), in collaboration with the Food and Drug Administration (FDA), has developed ClinicalTrials.gov to provide up-to-date information for locating federally and privately supported clinical trials for a wide range of diseases and conditions. ClinicalTrials.gov currently contains more than 100,000 research trials sponsored by the NIH, other federal agencies, and private industry. This Web site provides a wealth of information about cancer research and can help you to understand how clinical trials work, and the potential risks and benefits. The site presents research results and includes many links to other agencies and resources including a guide to understanding genetic conditions and the U.S. National Library of Medicine.

My Family Health Portrait
https://familyhistory.hhs.gov

My Family Health Portrait was developed in collaboration between the Office of the Surgeon General and the National Human Genome Research Institute. This Web-based tool helps users organize family health history information and then print it out for presentation to their health care provider. In addition, the tool helps users save their family history information to their own computer and even share family history information with other family members. The tool is free to all users. No user information is saved on any computer of the U.S. government. After entering family history information, the Family Health Portrait tool will create and print out a graphical representation of your family's generations and the health disorders that may have moved from one generation to the next. That is a powerful tool for predicting diseases for which you may be at risk. Your health care provider can help you make use of this information. If you prefer to use a paper version of the tool to gather and record your family information, printable PDFs are available in several languages.

Office of Cancer Complementary and Alternative Medicine
www.cancer.gov/cam

The Office of Cancer Complementary and Alternative Medicine (OCCAM) was established to improve the quality of care of cancer patients, as well as those at risk for cancer and those recovering from cancer treatment, by contributing to the advancement of evidence-based complementary and alternative medicine (CAM) and the sciences that support it. This government office encourages collaboration between cancer researchers and CAM practitioners through lectures, conferences, and workshops. The office also identifies gaps in existing cancer CAM research and creates funding opportunities to increase the number of high quality studies on this topic, as well as providing an expert review of CAM contents on behalf of NCI for institute-supported projects and programs.

National Cancer Institute
www.cancer.gov

The National Cancer Institute (NCI) is part of the National Institutes of Health (NIH) and is the federal government's principal agency for cancer research and training. The NCI conducts and supports research, training, health information dissemination, and other programs with respect to the cause, diagnosis, prevention, and treatment of cancer, rehabilitation from cancer, and the continuing care of cancer patients and their families. The NCI Web site provides information about all types of cancer, clinical trials research, cancer statistics, research funding, and publications of research results, among many other topics. A large number of valuable links are available on the NCI Web site.

Within the NCI is the Office of Cancer Centers that is responsible for designating sixty-six nationwide Comprehensive Cancer Centers, which are characterized by strong organizational capabilities, institutional commitment, and trans-disciplinary, cancer-focused science, in addition to experienced scientific and administrative leadership, and state-of-the-art cancer research and patient care facilities. A list of Comprehensive Cancer Centers can be found on this Web site.

U.S. Food and Drug Administration
www.fda.gov

The U.S. Food and Drug Administration (FDA) is an agency within the Department of Health and Human Services that is responsible for protecting the public health by assuring the safety, efficacy, and security of drugs, biological products, medical devices, our nation's food supply, cosmetics, and products that emit radiation, and by regulating the manufacture, marketing, and distribution of tobacco products.

The FDA is also responsible for advancing public health by helping to speed innovations that make medicines and foods more effective, safer, and more affordable; and by helping the public obtain accurate, science-based information on medicines and foods, and on reducing tobacco use to improve health.

Diagnostic Company Resources—For Profit

Agendia
www.agendia.com

Agendia has developed a gene signature assay known as Blue Print that separates breast cancer into into three types: (1) luminal, (2) basal, and (3) Her2.

In addition, they have developed an RT-PCR assay known as Target Print that determines estrogen, progesterone, and Her2-positivity.

Agendia has also developed a molecular diagnostic test called MammaPrint that can help to predict the risk of breast cancer recurrence in the first five years after diagnosis. MammaPrint gives physicians a tool to help separate "high" risk from "low" risk early-stage breast cancer patients and better gauge "high" risk patients' need for chemotherapy.

Caris Life Sciences
www.carislifesciences.com

Caris Life Sciences has developed a test to examine the genetic and molecular makeup that is unique to each patient's tumor. By comparing the tumor's information with data from clinical studies from thousands of the world's leading cancer researchers, Caris can help the physician determine which treatments are likely to be most effective and which treatments are likely to be ineffective for each patient.

Genomic Health

www.genomichealth.com

Genomic Health is a molecular diagnostics company that is committed to improving the quality of cancer treatment through the development of genomic-based testing. The diagnostic tests, Oncotype DX breast cancer assay and Oncotype DX colon cancer assay, generate information that health care providers and patients can use in making decisions about treatment options. The Oncotype DX breast cancer assay is a test that examines a patient's tumor tissue and gives information about a particular patient's disease that can help individualize breast cancer treatment planning and identify options. Learn more about the Oncotype DX breast cancer assay on the Genomic Health Web site described above or by visiting www.oncotypeDX.com.

Myriad Genetics, Inc.

www.myriad.com

Myriad Genetics is a molecular diagnostic company that has developed tests to help identify genetic variations that are the most common causes of inherited cancers. These tests assist doctors and patients to understand the genetic basis of human disease and the role that genes play in the onset, progression, and treatment of disease. The Myriad Genetics Web site includes an online family cancer history tool and a hereditary cancer quiz that can help patients to evaluate their hereditary cancer risk.

Rational Therapeutics Cancer Laboratories

www.rational-t.com

Rational Therapeutics uses a patient's tumor tissue to test against a number of standard chemotherapies, and where possible, the newest targeted agents. Typically, the laboratory uses living tumor cells collected during biopsy or surgery and analyzes the response to individual drugs or a combination of drugs.

Weisenthal Cancer Group

www.weisenthalcancer.org

The Weisenthal Cancer Group provides a laboratory-testing method called Functional Tumor Cell Profiling. Functional Cell Profiling is a personalized medicine approach that tests a patient's living cancer cells against a broad array of anticancer drugs and drug combinations. Functional Cell Profiling identifies—for each patient—the specific treatment that offers the highest probability of treatment success.

Dr. John Link's Web site

drjohnlinkbreastcancercare.com

With the publication of the fifth edition of *The Breast Cancer Survival Manual* I decided to create a Web site to serve as a companion to the manual so that women will have continuous access to new information and services available for breast cancer care. Because the information presented in each of the editions is only current as of the day of publication, I felt it was essential to provide immediate access to new innovations that can help patients to survive and survive well! My goal is to continue to educate and empower all breast cancer survivors with tools that will aid in their journey. On this Web site you will find access to the electronic medical records application that you can use to help store and manage your personal health records. You will also find detailed information on how to request a second opinion. The Web site also includes links to new technology, services, and information essential for all breast cancer survivors. I hope that you visit this site often and that along with this manual your personal journey is made easier.

Glossary

Abraxane: Albumin-covered paclitaxel (Taxol).

acute: Sharp, intense, and of short duration.

adjuvant: Auxiliary, an aid to remove or prevent disease.

amino acids: The building blocks of proteins and the end products of protein digestion.

ancillary: Additional, auxiliary.

angiogenesis: Development of blood vessels.

areola: A circular pigmented area around the breast nipple.

assay: Analysis of a substance.

atypical lobular hyperplasia: Abnormally shaped cells proliferating excessively in the normal tissue arrangement of a breast lobule. Also called lobular neoplasia, type I.

autosomal dominant gene: Non-sex-based gene that requires only one copy in order to be expressed.

autosomal recessive gene: Non-sex-based gene that requires two copies in order to be expressed.

axillary lymph nodes: Lymph nodes in the armpit.

basal type: A breast cancer type in the new classification based on genetic analysis. Also called triple-negative.

basement membrane: The separating membrane that provides a boundary from adjacent tissue.

biopsy: Excision of a small piece of living tissue for microscopic examination; usually performed to establish a diagnosis.

BRCA1: First discovered hereditary breast cancer gene mutation.

BRCA2: Second discovered hereditary breast cancer gene mutation.

chronic: Of long duration.

clear margin: Surrounding area of tissue that is clear of cancer cells after surgery.

colloid cancer: A rare ductal cancer also known as mucinous cancer.

combination chemotherapy: Combining drugs together in a single treatment.

cribriform: A pattern of cancer cell growth inside the breast duct that resembles mesh.

cystosarcoma phyllodes: A tumor of the breast that is of nonepithelial origin.

cytotoxic agents: Chemicals that destroy cells or prevent their multiplication.

differentiation: Cancer cells can be well, moderately, or poorly differentiated. The degree of differentiation describes how closely the cancer cell remains in appearance to a normal healthy cell. Well-differentiated cancer cells most closely resemble a normal cell, while poorly differentiated cells look least like normal cells and are therefore more malignant.

disease: The lack (*dis*) of ease; a pathological condition of the body.

DNA repair gene: A gene responsible for repairing DNA. A mutation in a DNA repair gene can lead to cancer. PARP is one example of a DNA repair gene.

dose dense: Intensifying the administration of chemotherapy by shortening the time interval between treatments.

ductal cancer in situ (DCIS): A cancer encapsulated within the breast ducts.

ductal cell: A cell from the duct of the breast.

electron beam boost: Use of radioactive particles to target a specific area of the body with additional radiation treatments.

enzyme: An organic catalyst produced by living cells but capable of acting independently. Enzymes produce chemical changes without being changed themselves.

epithelium: Cells that form a barrier to underlying tissue such as skin, ducts, and glands.

estrogen: The female sex hormone produced by the ovary. Estrogens are responsible for the development of secondary sexual characteristics and for cyclic changes in the vaginal epithelium and endothelium of the uterus.

excision: Surgical removal by cutting.

excisional biopsy: A biopsy in which an entire lesion is removed.

expander: A polyurethane flexible implant that is placed under the tissue and is enlarged manually by inserting a fluid, usually saline.

first-generation prognostic factors: Simple validated measures for predicting outcomes that have proved their usefulness in the past.

free radicals: Damage to tissue by molecules containing an odd number of electrons.

genistein: A phytoestrogen produced by soy products.

Her2 oncogene: An oncogene that is abnormally stimulated to produce an excess of protein, affecting cell division in the breast.

Herceptin: The brand name for trastuzumab, a drug that is used in Her2-positive breast cancer.

heterogeneous disease: A disease that does not manifest itself in the same way in every patient; having varying or dissimilar characteristics.

high-grade cancer: A cancer with a modified Bloom Richardson (BR) Grading Scale of 8 to 9, commonly with a high vascular component.

histologic grade: The microscopic measure and evaluation of the structure of a cancer.

homogeneous: Uniform in nature; a similar cause.

hormone: A substance that originates in a gland and is conveyed through the blood to another part of the body, stimulating it by chemical action to increase functional activity or increase secretion of other hormones.

hyperplasia: An increase in the number of cells in the lining of a gland.

hypothesis: An educated guess; a preliminary assumption based on enough observation to place it beyond mere speculation but requiring further experiments for verification.

infiltrating lobular carcinoma: Cancerous cells in the breast lobule that have spread through the basement membrane into the surrounding breast tissue.

in situ: In the normal place without disturbing the surrounding tissue, localized.

intraoperative radiation therapy (IORT): A form of breast irradiation administered as a single treatment during surgery.

invasive cancer: Cancer cells that penetrate the basement membrane, resulting in spread to healthy tissue.

isoflavone: A chemical found in soy products.

lobular carcinoma in situ (LCIS): A change in the breast lobule that increases the risk of breast cancer. It is a marker for breast cancer. The new nomenclature is lobular neoplasia, type 2.

lobular cell: A cell in the lobule of the breast; used for making milk.

lobular neoplasia: An abnormal accumulation of cells in the terminal lobule. When present, increases the risk of future breast cancer. Previously called LCIS.

local control: The control of cancer in the breast.

local recurrence: The return of cancerous cells to the breast.

luminal type: A type of breast cancer cell in the new breast cancer classification based on genetic analysis.

lumpectomy: Surgical removal of a tumor from the breast to clear margins not including the lymph nodes. Also known as a wide local excision.

lymphedema: Edema or swelling caused by obstruction of lymph channels.

lymph node: A rounded body consisting of an accumulation of lymphatic tissue found at intervals in the course of lymphatic vessels. Lymph nodes vary in size from a pinhead to an olive and can occur singularly or in groups. They produce lymphocytes and monocytes, and serve to filter matter from entering the bloodstream.

macroscopic: Visible to the naked eye; gross observation.

main tumor: A spontaneous new growth of tissue made up of abnormally dividing cells that form a mass.

markers: Tumor antigens that can be measured by blood tests.

mastectomy: See simple mastectomy; skin-sparing mastectomy.

mastitis: Inflammation or infection of the breast.

MBR scale: Modified Bloom-Richardson grading of the degree of malignancy.

metastatic disease: Movement of cancer cells from one part of the body to another.

microinvasion: Invasion of cancer cells through the breast duct into adjacent tissue at a microscopic level.

mitosis: The reproduction of cells; the process of cell division.

mitotic rate: Rate or speed of cell division.

mutation: Any basic alteration in form, quality, or some other characteristic. A change in genetic material of a chromosome that produces a new individual unlike its parents.

necrosis: Death of areas of tissue surrounded by healthy tissue.

neoadjuvant chemotherapy: The use of chemotherapy prior to curative surgery for local control.

neuropathy: Disease or damage of the nerves, causing lack of sensitivity or numbness.

oncogene: A gene that has the ability to induce a cell to become malignant. In addition to genes that induce tumor formation, there are antioncogenes that suppress tumors.

oncoplastic: Use of plastic and reconstructive techniques combined with oncologic surgery.

palpable: Capable of being touched or felt.

papillary cancer: A type of ductal cancer in the breast.

pathology report: An evaluation performed by a physician who specializes in the diagnosis of structural and functional changes in tissue that result from disease processes.

pedicle: A stem of tissue containing blood vessels allowing for the movement of that tissue to another area of the body.

perimenopausal: Around menopause.

phytochemicals: Chemicals found in plants.

phytoestrogen: An estrogen-like substance produced by plants.

pilot studies: Research investigations that explore a particular drug, technique, or idea.

placebo: Inactive substance given to patients as medicine; also used in control studies of drugs.

polyunsaturated fats: Fats made up of long-chain carbon compounds with many carbon atoms joined by double or triple bonds.

premalignant: Before metastasis; cancerous growth (as in lobular neoplasia).

progesterone: A steroid hormone from the corpus luteum and placenta. It is responsible for changes in the endometrium in the second half of the menstrual cycle, development of the maternal placenta, and development of the mammary glands.

prognosis: Estimated chance of recovery from the disease or chance that the disease will recur.

proliferate: To grow or multiply by rapidly producing new cells; to increase or spread at a rapid rate.

prophylactic: Contributing to the prevention of infection or disease.

quadrant: One-quarter; the breast is divided into four quadrants: upper outer, upper inner, lower outer, and lower inner.

randomized clinical trial: An investigation of the effects of a drug administered to human subjects. The goal is to define the clinical efficiency and pharmacological effects (toxicity, side effects, interactions) of the substance. This is done by a random method of assigning subjects to experimental treatment or nontreatment groups.

receptor: A cell component that combines with a drug, hormone, or chemical mediator to alter the function of the cell.

reconstruction: The action of constructing again. In breast reconstruction, the surgically altered breast is returned to its approximate original state.

recurrence: Return of the cancer.

remission: The period when cancer appears to be inactive.

satellite nodules: Small structures attached to the larger tumor.

sensitivity: The ability to react to stimuli. The value of a diagnostic test; the procedure of clinical observation.

sentinel node: The first lymph node draining a malignant tumor.

sequential chemotherapy: Using drugs in a singular manner, in a set sequence.

SERDs: Selective estrogen receptor downregulators.

SERMs: Selective estrogen receptor modulators.

simple mastectomy: Removal of the entire breast, leaving the adjacent lymph nodes and chest muscles intact. Also called a total mastectomy.

simulation: Radiation planning session designed to map out the radiation field.

skin-sparing mastectomy: A mastectomy that spares most of the skin overlying the removed breast tissue that can then be filled with tissue from a transfer or silicone or saline implant.

sporadic: Occurring occasionally or at scattered intervals.

stage: Denoting diagnosis and treatment on the basis of observation, pathology, and symptoms of patients.

staging system: The assessment of a cancer by size and quality.

state of the art: The best treatment available.

systemic control: The control of cancer throughout the body.

systemic spread: The spread of cancer cells to other organs via the bloodstream.

taxane: A class of chemotherapy drugs.

tissue transfer: Breast reconstruction by removing tissue from other parts of the body and replacing it in the breast.

toxicity: The extent or degree of being poisonous.

transverse rectus abdominis myocutaneous (TRAM) flap: Breast reconstruction surgery that uses tissue from the abdomen to rebuild the breast.

tubular cancer: A slow-growing, rare type of ductal cancer.

tumor: A growth of abnormal cells that forms a mass or lump. This can be benign or malignant.

tumor suppressor gene: A protective gene that normally limits the growth of tumors. When there is a mutation in a tumor suppressor gene it may fail to keep a cancer from growing. BRCA1 is an example of a tumor suppressor gene.

vascular system: The heart, blood vessels, lymphatics, and their parts considered collectively.

well-differentiated: Cancer cells that closely resemble the normal cells from which they developed.

wide local excision (WLE): See lumpectomy.

Index

Page numbers in *italics* refer to illustrations.

About the Author

DR. JOHN LINK is recognized as one of the world's leading breast cancer specialists. As the pioneer developer of Breastlink Medical Group, he established one of the first comprehensive breast care centers in the United States based on his innovative "optimal care" model that incorporates all aspects of screening, diagnosis, treatment, and follow-up within a single medical environment. Using this model, thousands of women from around the world have benefited from Dr. Link's philosophy that it is possible to provide women with individualized care tailored to their unique cancer situation using a team approach. By bringing all of the treating specialties together in one location patients can feel confident that their treatment team is coordinated and working together to provide the very best care available.

Dr. Link was born in San Diego, California, and has spent his career practicing medicine in Southern California. He attended the University of Southern California (USC) for undergraduate studies where he was an Academic All American. As a gifted runner and captain of the USC track team Dr. Link held a world record in the two-mile relay (4 × 880). When his beloved track coach was diagnosed with cancer and died at the age of 42, Dr. Link knew that he wanted to pursue medicine and dedicate his career to the care and treatment of cancer patients. While at the USC

School of Medicine he chose medical oncology as his focus and after graduation he decided to specialize exclusively in breast cancer.

With the publication of this 5th edition of *The Breast Cancer Survival Manual*, Dr. Link continues to emphasize the importance of educating breast cancer patients about their disease and the different treatment options available so that they can be active participants in the development of their treatment plan. He believes all women should be empowered to survive this disease and that by understanding the risks and benefits of different treatment options women will feel confident in the choices they make. Dr. Link's philosophy is that women should not only survive breast cancer, but they should survive well, and through careful evaluation and planning women can receive optimal care for their unique situations.

In addition to his active medical practice, Dr. Link travels and lectures about breast cancer diagnosis and treatment to community groups, medical oncologists and other specialists, medical students, professional organizations, and private industry. The first edition of the *Breast Cancer Survival Manual* was published in 1998 and since that time Dr. Link has contributed to numerous journal articles, poster sessions, and book chapters on breast cancer.

Dr. Link and his wife Nancy have six children and live in Southern California where they enjoy golf, travel, and collecting contemporary art. To learn more about Dr. Link and his optimal care plan for breast cancer please visit: www.drjohnlink.com.